Mina Carson

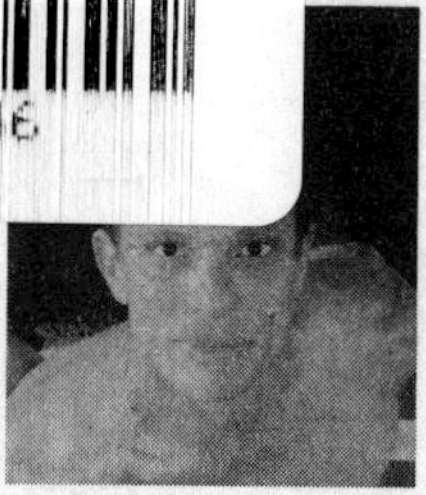

Briana Coiner

STUART RAY SARBACKER and KEVIN KIMPLE

THE EIGHT LIMBS OF YOGA

STUART RAY SARBACKER is an associate professor of comparative religion and Indian philosophy at Oregon State University in Corvallis, Oregon. His academic work is centered on the theory and practice of yoga in the traditions of Hinduism, Buddhism, and Jainism, and in its contemporary nonsectarian manifestations. He is the author of *Samādhi: The Numinous and Cessative in Indo-Tibetan Yoga* and of numerous scholarly articles on yoga. He has trained extensively in contemporary yoga and meditation traditions in India and the United States.

KEVIN KIMPLE is the founder and director of the Eugene School of Yoga in Eugene, Oregon, where he instructs daily in the Mysore-style setting. He is among a select group of practitioners to be personally authorized to teach Ashtanga Vinyasa Yoga by Sri K. Pattabhi Jois, after living in Mysore, India, for more than three years studying yoga, Sanskrit, philosophy, and music. A former professional dancer, Kimple toured extensively with the Martha Graham Ensemble, MOMIX, Bella Lewitzky, and other notable dance troupes. He received a black belt in Shaolin kung fu and has been teaching mind-body disciplines in intimate studio settings for the past twenty years. He is also an avid gardener and shares his experience and enthusiasm for life freely.

THE EIGHT LIMBS OF YOGA

THE EIGHT LIMBS OF YOGA

A HANDBOOK FOR LIVING YOGA PHILOSOPHY

STUART RAY SARBACKER and KEVIN KIMPLE

Foreword by Christopher Key Chapple

North Point Press
A division of Farrar, Straus and Giroux
New York

North Point Press
A division of Farrar, Straus and Giroux
18 West 18th Street, New York 10011

Printed in the United States of America
First edition, 2015

Library of Congress Cataloging-in-Publication Data
Sarbacker, Stuart Ray, 1969–
The eight limbs of yoga : a handbook for living yoga philosophy / Stuart Ray Sarbacker and Kevin Kimple ; foreword by Christopher Key Chapple.
pages cm
Includes bibliographical references.
ISBN 978-0-86547-768-1 (paperback) — ISBN 978-0-86547-769-8 (e-book)
1. Yoga—Philosophy. I. Kimple, Kevin. II. Title.

RA781.67 .S37 2015
613.7'046—dc23

2014039397

Designed by Jonathan D. Lippincott

www.fsgbooks.com
www.twitter.com/fsgbooks • www.facebook.com/fsgbooks

5 7 9 10 8 6 4

To all aspiring yogins and yoginīs

discipline

By the strength gained through this practice, we can come to know the method of bringing the mind and sense organs under control. Thus can we achieve yoga. For it is only through the control of the mind and sense organs that we come to know our true nature, and not through intellectual knowledge, or by putting on the garb of a yogi.

—Sri K. Pattabhi Jois, *Yoga Mala*

sexual misconduct?

If you see the Buddha on the road, kill him."

Contents

Foreword

This concise book provides a user's guide to the practice of yoga. Nearly twenty million people regularly practice some form of yoga in the United States. A typical yoga class will include some stretching, some yoga postures, focused breathing, and, generally at the end of the class, a period of deep relaxation. Yoga returns people to their bodies and breath, allowing for a contemplative space to arise.

In some yoga classes, students may be encouraged to pause and cultivate a moment of mindfulness, and perhaps carry that from the yoga class into the world. The beginning point of being mindful, as this book gently shows, entails being aware of the basic need for inner and outer safety. Yoga advocates the principle of do no harm. By restraining oneself from aggression or violence in thought, word, and deed, one develops an atmosphere of peace that can put others at ease. This principle then governs the other ethical teachings of yoga: to be truthful, honest, respectful in matters of sexuality, and nonhoarding. With this ongoing discipline, a person can then seek the positive yoga components of purity, happiness, steadfastness, contemplative study, and dedication to higher ideals.

The mind states of yoga result in the ability to gather oneself inward, to cultivate focus. This focus can lead to meditation, the capacity to sustain attention on a goal higher than and beyond self-concern. Building on the traditional philosophy known as Sāṃkhya, yoga provides techniques by which one can rise above mistaken notions governed by ignorance, egoism, attraction, repulsion, and the drive toward self-perpetuation. By understanding the workings of the realm of karma, and by reshaping the body and mind through mastery of breath, one can distinguish between the realm of change and the changeless witness. This witness consciousness, a place of freedom, can become, through yoga, the ground for integrative being in the world.

Samādhi, the goal of yoga, allows one to dissolve the boundaries between self and world. This experience takes many forms and can involve many different techniques. Yoga leaves open many options and can be practiced by atheists as well as by devotees of one of the many embodiments of the divine. By focusing on how the mind functions, yoga shows what is possible, without demanding allegiance to any one particular set of beliefs. Buddhists, Hindus, Jainas, Sikhs, and Muslims have used yogic techniques for centuries, techniques that are now being widely applied in the modern world by Christians, Jews, and secularists.

This book, remarkable for its brevity, provides a road map for the exploration of yoga. Stuart Ray Sarbacker and Kevin Kimple have masterfully covered the basics of yoga philosophy without compromising its complexity and profundity. Read in conjunction with one of the many good translations of Patañjali's *Yogasūtra*, this book can help the student of yoga understand the transformative potential of yoga practice.

Christopher Key Chapple
Doshi Professor of Indic and Comparative Theology
Director, Master of Arts in Yoga Studies
Loyola Marymount University

insight vs. integration

> James Boag

THE
EIGHT LIMBS
OF
YOGA

Introduction

The goal of this short book is to provide a concise and pragmatic guide to the application of the eight-limbed yoga (*aṣṭāṅgayoga*) in everyday life. The eight-limbed system is a clear and coherent framework that one can return to again and again to deepen and expand one's understanding and practice of yoga. In the *Yogasūtra* of Patañjali, a key text on Hindu yoga philosophy, the eight limbs are used to demonstrate the central principles of yoga, drawing together a spectrum of practices of self-discipline from Hindu, Buddhist, and Jaina sources. The eight limbs of yoga represent various forms of practice (*abhyāsa*) that move from the tangible outer world and the body to the subtle inner world of the mind. Progression through the limbs is a movement from external to internal, from social life to psychological life, rooted in the realization that our lives "out in the world" and our inner lives are connected and coextensive in important ways. The various yoga traditions of India have all recognized the great potential for self-transformation through yoga practice, whether it is thought of in terms of worldly power, liberation from suffering, or some combination of the two. All recognize that to transform oneself through yoga is to transform one's relationship with the world in profound ways.

In the context of Indian philosophical and religious traditions, yoga is understood to transform the body and mind in such a way that one's capacities for action and perception are enhanced. This enhancement is the basis for legendary "yoga powers" that are discussed in the literature of yoga, such as the *Yogasūtra*, using the language of "spiritual accomplishment" (*siddhi*). These abilities include reading others' minds, heightened powers of vision and hearing, and magical flight, among others. Whether we understand these powers literally or as metaphors, the message is clear: yoga leads to a transformation of the human person such that the limits of human experience are extended and human abilities are perfected. Yet these powers or capacities are often represented in the literature of yoga as impediments or even temptations that may distract a yoga practitioner from the pursuit of liberating knowledge, which is held to be a superior spiritual goal. The idea of pursuing yoga, or any ascetic discipline, for the sake of power is by no means foreign to the Indian philosophical and religious context. In fact, the narratives of Hinduism, Buddhism, and Jainism are filled with examples of individuals who attained great power through yogic and ascetic practice and yet wielded that power in a less than enlightened manner.

In the *Yogasūtra*, such power is acknowledged as real, but the exercise of power out of greed and other afflicted emotions is understood to lead to future misery and the loss of any peace or equanimity that had been found in the practice. The peace or equanimity that one obtains through seeing things clearly is valued above and beyond egocentric aspirations to obtain worldly power and control over others. As we will see later, this is part of the reason why the first limb of yoga is moral restraint (*yama*). Only a person whose practice is rooted in nonviolence, truthfulness, nonstealing, sexual restraint, and nongreed will be able to manage the power, and thus the potential threat, that comes out of the accomplishments to be found in the practice of yoga. In the system of Patañjali, yoga is about obtaining freedom from identification with worldly objects and resting in a state of peace that is beyond the flux of psychophysical (mental and physical) life. This peace is an internal freedom from the mental and physical pain of embodied life, and it lays a foundation upon which to build a life that is rooted in peace and of benefit to others.

1

What Is Yoga?

YS I.14 *sa tu dīrghakālanairantaryasatkārāsevito dṛḍhabhūmiḥ*
It [practice] becomes grounded firmly when dwelled upon for an extended time with dedication and without interruption.

Yoga means something akin to "yoking" or "joining." It is derived from a Sanskrit word that was used in its early contexts as the term for joining a cart or chariot to an animal, such as a horse or an ox. Yoga, in this sense, is a discipline that brings physical and psychic (mental) life under control for the purpose of spiritual development. In ancient Hindu literature, the skillful control of a horse and chariot often served as a symbol for this type of spiritual discipline and as a metaphor for spiritual mastery. Just as a physically unskilled charioteer is at the mercy of the power and force of the horses, a person who is spiritually undisciplined will be at the mercy of habit and the senses. As a skilled charioteer is able to drive a chariot with grace and ease, so too the spiritually disciplined person masters his or her body and mind and is able to accomplish goals with grace and ease.

This is accomplished not through brute force but through the force of the refinement of body and mind.

Following this, yoga can be understood as a solution to the timeless problem of the "gap" between will and action. Though we may have clear ideas of what we hope to accomplish in our lives, we often struggle internally with ourselves and in some cases act as if we were our own worst enemy. Habits and desires drive us toward patterns of thought and action that are unproductive and at odds with our values and goals, leading to harm, guilt, and despair. Though we may be committed deeply to our moral or spiritual development, we often find that we cannot swim against the tide of our own personal history and the pull of moment-to-moment impulses. Yoga proposes one possible approach to this perennial problem—a method for disciplining body and mind that provides the steadiness and strength necessary for self-transcendence and growth beyond the boundaries of our habitual ways of thinking and acting. This is described in Buddhist meditation traditions as developing a flexibility, or pliancy, of mind and body. What this means is that through disciplining the body and developing a contemplative practice, the thoughts and habits that impede our ability to act with integrity and purpose are weakened or suppressed, and we are given a window of opportunity to shift our thoughts and habits in new directions, a heightened locus of control. We break out of the scattered, frustrated mode of everyday living and enter into a mode of thinking and acting in which our efforts are more willful, fruitful, and powerful. In other words, yoga provides a method for building integrity and willpower that allows us to overcome the inner and outer pulls of destructive habit energy in our everyday lives, and it allows us to cultivate habits that are constructive.

In the *Yogasūtra*, yoga is presented as both the goal and the method of spiritual practice. Yoga is defined at the beginning of the text as *cittavṛttinirodha*, which is often translated as the "cessation of mental fluctuations." It is also shown to be the method whereby this cessation (*nirodha*) is brought about. The eight-limbed yoga (*aṣṭāṅgayoga*) is the system of practice that brings a practitioner from purification to illumination and upward to a state of complete peace. A key commentator on the *Yogasūtra*, Vyāsa, asserts that yoga can also be identified with *samādhi*, or deep meditative contemplation. In other words, through the practice of yoga, there is the experience of deep serenity and clarity, an ability to rest in a state of self-collected peace without being swept up and caught up in the activity of the mind, body, or world. A popular Zen Buddhist saying relates this idea with respect to the reflection of the moon in water—when the waves of the lake have settled, the scattered reflection of the moon is drawn together into a coherent and clear image, and there is a reflection of undistorted reality. When the turbulence of the mind, manifested in various forms of mental activity, has settled down like the water's waves, clarity and integrity manifest and there is an experience of freedom.

Cessation of mental fluctuation, according to Patañjali, is brought about by two complementary principles of spiritual life, namely, practice (*abhyāsa*) and dispassion (*vairāgya*). These two principles represent the dynamic relationship at the heart of yogic discipline. This dynamic is between the forces of effort and detachment, where some things are to be taken up and others given up. Most of us can recognize situations in our own lives where these principles are playing out or have played out—situations in which we find ourselves negotiating between active participation in making something happen and letting go and letting things run their course. As we have pursued athletic, literary, or musical interests or careers, we have recognized the ways in which physical and mental development are tied into our dedicated efforts and our willingness to make sacrifices in order to have the time and energy to accomplish our goals. On a more subtle level, many of us have also experienced the dynamic relationship between pushing ourselves to high performance and recognizing our limits—the need to counterbalance effort with restorative inaction for the sake of recovery. This dynamic of practice and dispassion might be one of the most valuable philosophical concepts in the yoga tradition with respect to the greater parameters of one's life. We are subject to flux in our lives, wavelike rhythms of change that call for different responses at different times. The practice of modern postural forms of yoga creates familiarity with the cycles of energy, strength, and flexibility that encourage us to respond by practicing with appropriate degrees of vigor and patient ease. Meditative or contemplative practices may involve the conscious cultivation of particular meditation objects and attitudes one day, and a more receptive and dispassionate dealing with emotions or other experiences on another day. Yoga as such is not a singular approach but represents a range of responses to the changing conditions of mind, body, and environment. The basic dynamic of practice and dispassion demonstrates the validity and value of both activity and detachment as appropriate responses at different moments in practice and in life. This dynamic is intuitive for many people and is also found in various philosophical and religious contexts. The so-called Serenity Prayer encapsulates a similar way of approaching spiritual life—roughly as changing what one can change, accepting what one cannot change, and having the wisdom to know the difference. For Patañjali, practice becomes successful when it is applied consistently and energetically for an extended period of time, persevering through the ups and downs of life. Dispassion, or nonattachment, is considered perfected when no desire arises for either material or spiritual objects, a freedom from being bound to any worldly object of desire.

In yoga philosophy, practitioners of yoga are encouraged to cultivate faith (*śraddhā*), energy (*vīrya*), mindfulness (*smṛti*), contemplation (*samādhi*), and wisdom (*prajñā*), with the understanding that the more ardent and intense the level of practice, the closer the practitioner is to his or her goal. A technique that is highlighted as being uniquely fruitful in the practice of yoga is the "Dedication to the Lord" (*īśvarapraṇidhāna*), which refers to dedication and devotion to the ideal *yogin* or *yoginī*. Īśvara is portrayed as a master of yoga who has never been bound by the fluctuations of the mind and who serves as the archetype or model for the condition of spiritual realization. Commentators on this section of Patañjali's yoga refer to *īśvarapraṇidhāna* as a form of devotion (*bhakti*), a passionate or emotion-infused attitude of reverence for this deity—a god, or even God, who exemplifies the nature of a person in the liberated state. The principal method of *īśvarapraṇidhāna* is the recitation of the mantra syllable OṂ, which is understood to be the representation of the sound, or speech, of Īśvara. Through meditation on the OṂ, the obstacles to concentration are removed, and *samādhi* is perfected in an accelerated fashion. It is not surprising, then, that OṂ should have a privileged place in yoga practice; it is understood to be the closest thing to a shortcut to spiritual development and realization in the yoga philosophy.

Contemplative practice, exemplified in the meditative state of *samādhi*, is understood in Patañjali's yoga to be a progressive process. As serenity of mind and concentration develop, mental activity becomes progressively more subtle, and the obstacles to spiritual development—such as fatigue, torpor, confusion, emotional instability, and the inability to concentrate—wane. One might choose a particular meditation object that suits one's mental temperament, such as the mantra OṂ, friendliness or compassion, the breath, or an inspiring spiritual figure. The various meditative objects have a common set of goals—reducing the effect of obstacles to spiritual progress and developing a deep and penetrating mental focus. According to Patañjali, as one develops the power of concentration, the mind becomes clear like a radiant jewel, and successive levels of deepening contemplation follow. These levels of contemplation move away from the intellectual or verbal modes of thinking toward a mode of concentration that is increasingly subtle, direct, and profound. As this deep meditative state reaches its limit, it is said that the fluctuations of the experience of the world, such as thought and sensation, become profoundly still, to the point at which a state of unshakable, mountainlike calm is achieved. According to Patañjali, the ultimate trajectory of such meditative processes is the attainment of a state of freedom in which no seeds of future suffering exist. In other words, as the process of meditation becomes perfected, the very roots of mental fluctuation are removed, and the practitioner enters into a state of self-sustaining peace, no longer subject to the highs and lows of embodied existence.

The Eight-Limbed Yoga (*Aṣṭāṅgayoga*)

The principal method for achieving the cessation (*nirodha*) of mental fluctuations, as illustrated by Patañjali in the second part of the *Yogasūtra*, is the practice of *aṣṭāṅgayoga*, or the "eight-limbed yoga." The second part of the *Yogasūtra* is entitled *sādhanapāda*, which means the "section on practice." Patañjali outlines a system of yogic practice that is characterized by eight parts, which represent a progression of yogic practice from the concrete and external to the subtle and internal aspects of human life. The limbs themselves are restraint (*yama*), observance (*niyama*), posture (*āsana*), breath control (*prāṇāyāma*), withdrawal (*pratyāhāra*), fixation (*dhāraṇā*), meditation (*dhyāna*), and contemplation (*samādhi*). *Yama* is further divided into five parts: nonharming (*ahiṃsā*), truthfulness (*satya*), nonstealing (*asteya*), sexual restraint (*brahmacarya*), and nongreed (*aparigraha*). *Niyama* is divided into five parts as well: cleanliness (*śauca*), contentment (*saṃtoṣa*), self-discipline (*tapas*), self-study (*svādhyāya*), and dedication to the lord (*īśvarapraṇidhāna*). The components of *yama* represent a reorientation to the social world, and those of *niyama* to the practitioner's body and spiritual life. *Yama* and *niyama*, as we will discuss at length later, provide the larger frame of meaning in which the discipline of yoga is performed. The limbs of *āsana*, *prāṇāyāma*, and *pratyāhāra* represent a mastery of physical form, of energy, and of the senses. The limbs of *dhāraṇā*, *dhyāna*, and *samādhi* represent a progression from the very beginning of developing concentration to the deep meditative absorption or contemplation of *samādhi*. Together these last three constitute yogic mastery (*saṃyama*). The first five limbs together are referred to as the outer limbs (*bahiraṅga*) of yoga in that they represent a range of experience from the social world to the operation of the senses. The final three are referred to as the inner limbs (*antaraṅga*), which focus on the mind and culminate in the attainment of yogic mastery and, ultimately, liberation.

The progression from concrete to subtle moves from the experience of everyday life, including interactions with others, through the individual's body and then ultimately to the most subtle aspects of mind. This notion of a progression of steps in this practice is sometimes likened to the idea of a ladder of yoga practices, or a series of steps that are sequential in nature. In this analysis, the *yama* and *niyama* practices establish the foundation—through cultivating a peaceful, detached mode of existence and a spiritual discipline, one prepares oneself for the physical and mental exertions of yoga. With the establishment of *āsana*, one has a level of comfort and stability in the body that is conducive to contemplation; likewise, the control of breath prepares a person energetically and mentally for contemplative practice. The withdrawal of the senses from their objects yields a fertile ground for developing concentration. The inner limbs of yoga—fixation, meditation, and contemplation—then focus and deepen concentration until it reaches a state of fruitful perfection.

Another valid way to look at the relationship between the limbs is as a sort of wheel with many spokes that mutually reinforce one another. From this perspective, every limb of yoga supports the others. Just as it might be said that the practice of *ahiṃsā*, or nonharming, and the peaceful life it entails provide for the development of the mental calm of meditation, it could be said that the mental calm of meditation might help dissolve angry thoughts that lead to harming others. Similarly, the development of a stable and comfortable posture and the regulation of breath might be said to contribute to both mental clarity and to a lessening of feelings of greed, craving, and so on. It is not uncommon for teachers of modern yoga traditions that focus on *āsana* to state that all of the eight limbs of yoga can be mastered within the practice of *āsana*. Or, alternately, some teachers will state that though *āsana* is the third limb of the *aṣṭāṅgayoga* system, it is in fact practiced first.

If we look at the issue of progression versus interrelation more closely, we can draw out a great lesson about the potential of this system as a dynamic mode of practice. One way to approach the eight limbs from a pragmatic point of view is to practice them sequentially. In other words, at any moment—dedicated to the practice of yoga or otherwise—one can use the eight-limb paradigm as a tool for self-reflection and the application of yoga practice. One can contemplate the ways in which the various limbs can be applied progressively to one's present condition, beginning with restraint (*yama*) and working up to contemplation (*samādhi*). One might also set up a more formal spiritual practice, beginning by attempting to observe the practice of moral restraint in one's life, perhaps especially in those places set aside for spiritual practice in the home or elsewhere. Building on this, a practitioner of yoga might dedicate him- or herself to the components of *niyama* through observing personal cleanliness, contentment, and self-discipline, through efforts to read and recite yoga texts, and through dedication to the personified spiritual ideal of yoga, Īśvara, either in abstract or concrete form. The practice of *niyama* as such might be further amplified through dedicating time and space to practicing its components, along with building relationships that help foster the practice of *yama* and *niyama* by means of the reinforcement of shared values. *Āsana* and *prāṇāyāma* are perhaps the most widely known and practiced of the eight limbs of yoga in the contemporary context, and so there are ample opportunities to study them with skilled teachers. Though there is less emphasis on meditation in many modern yoga traditions, it is a living part of some traditions, such as Transcendental Meditation, Satchidananda's Integral Yoga, and the contemporary Krishnamacharya tradition of T.K.V. Desikachar. A number of contemporary Buddhist traditions teach meditation practices that are related to Patañjali's system, as well, and they provide ample opportunities for both short-term and long-term meditation practice. When paired, home practice and formal institutional practice create a fruitful tension between personal and communal forms of engagement.

In addition to the establishment of a formal practice, in which one pursues the limbs over a relatively long duration of time, the eight limbs can be a touchstone for yoga within everyday life. In this respect, one can contemplate within any situation how the eight limbs would apply and how one might transform a given situation into an opportunity for spiritual practice. One might scan through the eight limbs sequentially, noting how a given life situation might call for the application of a particular limb. Likewise, the interrelated nature of the limbs means that whichever limb is appropriate, it will strengthen and provide for the practice of the others in their absence. The point here is that even the most mundane situations—such as grocery shopping, trivial encounters at work, taking kids to school—can be viewed as opportunities to practice yoga. The practice of *yama*, for example, has implications in virtually every social interaction.

Likewise, one might note how breath and posture are affected by the spectrum of experiences of everyday life. Perhaps most profound of all are the ways in which the moments of our lives are potentially sources of deep insight and contemplation, springing out of discerning alignment with the response that the world is calling for from moment to moment rather than being driven unconsciously to respond in unprofitable ways. According to one interpretation of the yoga philosophy, the same world that binds us to pain and misery, if understood properly, is the catalyst for our spiritual transformation and liberation. In other words, the same experiences that potentially bind us to misery can produce liberating insights into the nature of things, if we can properly reorient ourselves to them.

Living the Eight Limbs of Yoga

The following chapters are focused on bringing nuance and detail to the eight limbs of yoga and their application to everyday life and spiritual practice. The goal is to provide a practical guide for applying the principles of yoga to everyday life, in both formal and informal ways. It is intended to be a short and focused guide, one that can be read and reread to deepen one's understanding and experience of yoga as it applies to day-to-day existence and practice. It will serve as a reminder of what we have learned along the way and how we can keep that knowledge, and thus the practice of yoga, alive. Instead of focusing on the innumerable technical details of the philosophy of yoga, our focus will be on the pragmatic tools that yoga provides, which we hope will facilitate a new perspective on the world in a manner that unfolds naturally. We will encourage the reader to find ways to bridge the practice of yoga with other meaningful activities in life, allowing for a fruitful cross-pollination of the driving interests and commitments in one's life. In drawing together the concepts that are represented in the verses of the *Yogasūtra*, Patañjali brought together in his time a range of ideas and practices that were both traditional and innovative. Likewise, we believe that a living practice of yoga should not be static and fossilized but rather a dynamic, malleable discipline that can be continuously adapted to and connected to our modes of being in our world today. We also believe that a committed practice of yoga, rooted in the eight limbs, offers tremendous potential for self-transformation, for peace, and for building a more just and harmonious society.

2

Yama

RESTRAINT

YS II.31 *jātideśakālasamayānavacchinnāḥ sārvabhaumā mahāvratam*
When applied universally, not bound by conditions, time, place, or birth, it [moral restraint] is referred to as the "great vow."

Overview of *Yama*

Yama, or restraint, is the foundation of yoga practice as represented in the *aṣṭāṅgayoga* system of Patañjali. It represents the development of mastery over one's behavior, specifically with respect to one's relationship with other living beings. It is both a prerequisite for and an expression of spiritual liberation. To the degree that the observance of *yama* is seen as providing a foundation for bodily discipline and meditation, it could be said to be a preparatory practice. On the other hand, to the degree that *yama* represents an enlightened attitude reflected in everyday life, it might be seen as an expression of spiritual liberation in and of itself. The five *yama* practices—nonharming (*ahiṃsā*), truthfulness (*satya*), nonstealing (*asteya*), sexual restraint (*brahmacarya*), and nongreed (*aparigraha*)—can be viewed in the first sense as providing the peace, energy, and time required for spiritual practice. As long as a person is caught up in the emotional disturbance, energetic drain, and time-intensive nature of being consumed by their counterparts (e.g., harming others, lying, stealing, sexual obsession, and greediness), it is profoundly difficult to pursue the practice of yoga in a serious manner. It may be possible—certainly there are individuals who do not observe the *yama* precepts and yet are able to find the composure, time, and energy to practice—but on balance, and over time, practice will be difficult to sustain.

Not only do the elements of *yama* provide an ideal physical and mental environment for practice, they also help determine the longer-term trajectory of the practice by situating it within a sustainable and humane framework. Also, if yoga is viewed as a means of overcoming mental afflictions and disturbances, it makes intuitive sense that one would try to reduce conflict in one's larger life. Within some Buddhist traditions, arguably the most visible way that spiritual transformation becomes manifest in the world is in the form of moral transformation. In other words, not only is observance of a set of moral precepts the foundation for practice but spiritual liberation is evident in the perfection of such moral precepts. Spiritual liberation and moral transformation can be seen as coextensive, one not existing without the other.

The foundation of the five *yama* factors is, in a manner that is parallel to moral precepts in Buddhist and Jaina traditions, to be found in the first *yama* factor, nonharming (*ahiṃsā*). This factor, what Mohandas Gandhi referred to as "nonviolence," can be viewed as the axiomatic principle behind all of the moral precepts. In other words, the observance of truthfulness, nonstealing, sexual restraint, and nongreed keeps us from harming ourselves and others. The discernment of one's actions as harmful or not provides a basic moral principle that can be applied to any situation.

The practice of *yama*, and especially of *ahiṃsā*, points to a larger theme in Indian philosophical traditions regarding taking responsibility for one's moral legacy. A perfected person does not need yoga, or any practice for that matter, any longer. The practice of yoga is for imperfect people, especially those who are earnestly dedicated to transforming themselves and their moral and spiritual legacy in this world. As human beings we share a common experience of moral failings and regrets in our lives. Rather than conceiving of this as somehow a reason not to practice yoga, we can view these failings as a great motivating force for doing so with heightened intensity. Ideally, the energy of one's remorse or regret for personal failures can serve as fuel for the process of spiritual transformation. Instead of letting failure inhibit our practice, we can see it as a cause for renewed and redoubled effort. We can work to uproot the sources of our anger, greed, and so on, and in their place plant the seeds of future happiness for ourselves and those around us. From a Buddhist perspective, we should take up practice with zeal, recognizing how valuable every moment of our life is in coming to terms with what we have done in our lives and for setting ourselves on a profitable spiritual path. Acknowledging our failures, and cultivating an attitude that seeks out constructive ways to address our moral failings and to grow beyond them, is far superior to allowing them to destroy us and those around us. We can make amends to the degree possible, take responsibility, and dedicate ourselves to not repeating the same errors. This attitude itself is consistent with the overarching principle of *ahiṃsā*—that we should practice self-regulation with an eye to what is constructive, and we should avoid harmful attitudes and actions toward ourselves as well as others, letting go of self-destructive attitudes and behaviors.

Relative and Absolute Restraint

The *yama* factors encompass both the ideals of an inner spiritual practice and a commitment to a type of "good citizenship" within one's community. In Hindu, Buddhist, and Jaina traditions of yoga, a distinction is typically made between the observance of moral precepts in a relative manner versus an absolute one. Among householders, observation of these precepts is adapted to the realities of social life. The observation of sexual restraint, or *brahmacarya*, for example, is contextualized within the assumption that householders are not celibate. Therefore, the moral question is whether sexual relationships are consensual in nature and not marked by an imbalance of power or by physical or emotional abuse. Respect for social norms may be part of the larger picture for the householder with respect to these considerations, but it should be kept in mind that social norms may in fact condone certain types of harm, which appear "normal" due to their broad acceptance.

On the other hand, the practice of *brahmacarya* can also refer in an absolute way to the notion of the celibate religious student, either as a stage of life or as a chosen mode of living. In this case, the practitioner refrains from all expressions of sexual desire, and in doing so is said to preserve his or her physical vitality, in part through conserving the time and energy that would otherwise be directed toward this aspect of life. With respect to these approaches, relative and absolute, it can be said that each represents a different attitude toward the world, and each can be said to have a distinct set of values in the practice of yoga. The relative position is consistent with a world-affirming philosophy, and it might be said to have the benefit of testing one's commitment to observing the precepts and the practices. In other words, the "worldly" *yogin* or *yoginī* is forced to practice the principles of *yama* on an everyday basis, and it is quite clear to what degree the principles have been mastered. Anyone who has been in a long-term relationship, has children, or has everyday interactions with family, friends, or coworkers can understand how quickly one's sense of mastery over one's emotions and actions can break down as others push our buttons. These moments of disruption, where we face our own limitations—particularly with respect to the observance of *yama*—can be quite instructive as difficult but important opportunities to grow spiritually. Our responses to these moments are not only pivotal with respect to our own spiritual life but may well constitute one of the ways that we have a profound impact on others.

For the practitioner who has chosen renunciation of household life, the parameters are quite different. Separation from one's social world and one's material life into either a life of isolation or a spirituality-based community is a much more radical departure from everyday social life. One benefit, from a spiritual perspective, of doing so is that practicing in such a community provides an opportunity to invest oneself fully in intensive practice, with the distractions of everyday life at a minimum. Add to this the idea that one has access to teachers or even a whole community of people who have dedicated themselves to practice, and the appeal of such a lifestyle becomes very clear. The monastic traditions of Hinduism, Buddhism, and Jainism are all rooted in the notion that spiritual progress can be enhanced or accelerated through participation in intensive spiritual community. With respect to *yama*, if spiritual development is tied to moral development, then it makes sense to be part of a community that embodies those principles and makes it easier to observe them.

These paths each have their pitfalls. The householder may struggle to balance the commitment of time to his or her worldly pursuits and the time and energy demands of sustaining a serious practice, a struggle modern yoga practitioners often encounter, especially as they build families. The practitioner in isolation may never find his or her commitments tested in this way. However, the member of a spiritual community may find that the same habits of relationship, including issues of wealth and power, exist in a subtle or hidden form within an organization. It is also worth mentioning that these two paths might be said to represent a larger spectrum of possibilities rather than a basic, black-and-white choice. Many householder-practitioners attend workshops and retreats that allow them to practice in "ideal" environments for a temporary period. Likewise, many monastic practitioners teach at such retreats and interact with laypersons on a daily basis, thus having an ongoing connection with the everyday life of a larger community. It is worth mentioning that many of the key figures of modern yoga—such as Krishnamacharya and his disciples B.K.S. Iyengar and K. Pattabhi Jois—were householders. On the other hand, Swami Sivananda of Rishikesh and his disciple Swami Satchidananda are notable examples of the ongoing role of the renouncer paradigm in modern yoga traditions.

Ahiṃsā

The first member of *yama* is nonharming, or *ahiṃsā*. This is often understood, as mentioned above, to be at the root of the observance of all the moral precepts. In its most explicit sense, it refers to the idea of not physically harming, and especially not killing, humans, animals, or other living beings. It can have more subtle meanings, however, with respect to types of harm that are less visible or concrete, such as verbal violence that causes emotional harm to another individual or being. The most subtle of all are the ways in which thought itself may be of a harmful nature, even if it is not acted upon. One way to look at this is as a spectrum of harmful behavior that extends from the subtle or less tangible dimension of thought to the more concrete dimension of physical action. In Indian philosophical traditions, speech is often seen as a bridge between thought and physical action, an intermediate realm of action that is of unique importance from a moral standpoint. Some commentators on the yoga traditions use the terms *inner* observance versus *outer* observance to indicate the ways in which *ahiṃsā* is to be practiced. The inner dimension is the origin of the outer, and so ultimately the roots of violence are understood to be in the mind. However, it is often easier to begin with the restraint of the more concrete, visible actions that are the expression of thought than it is to work on thought directly. On the other hand, through disciplines like meditation, one can learn to be mindful of angry thoughts arising, and thus not be swayed by them. Also, one can cultivate attitudes that challenge such thinking when it arises, a concept that is sometimes referred to as applying meditative "antidotes" to thoughts of harm and so forth.

The observance of *ahiṃsā* has a number of intuitive applications, such as developing an attitude of kindness toward oneself and others. It is often asserted within traditions of yoga and meditation that a key part of being kind to others is developing that attitude first toward oneself, which goes along with the idea that being kind to others is an uphill battle at best if a person is unkind even to himself. To the degree that we are locked in an internal struggle with our own self-judgment and anger, we are going to have a difficult time engaging with others compassionately and practicing effectively. This is not to say that self-reflection or self-criticism is never warranted. Rather, the point is that an undue degree of aggression toward oneself is counterproductive to both one's own happiness and that of others.

Ahiṃsā may also call for rethinking one's lifestyle in important ways—such as becoming more mindful of diet and the ways in which it impacts other beings. For some this might mean a commitment to vegetarianism or veganism; for others it might be pursuing a diet in which the humane treatment of animals and the impact of farming on the environment are serious considerations. In the Indian tradition, Hindu, Buddhist, and Jaina practitioners have not fully agreed on what *ahiṃsā* means for their diets, and so they have applied the principle in different ways. However, they have all embraced the notion that one should bring awareness to one's consumption and be aware of the moral implications of one's diet. On another level, embracing the principle of *ahiṃsā* means bringing a mindful and conscious attitude to questions such as war, politics, economics, and many other dimensions of life where there are profound implications of a person's (and of a society's) actions with respect to the welfare of human and other forms of life. *Ahiṃsā* may call us to skillful action in the face of thinking and living patterns that promote harm and pain in our human communities and in the natural world. The discipline of yoga can provide the foundation of physical and psychic strength necessary for being an agent for change in the world. It is, in an ideal sense, a practice that works to help counter the self-perpetuating cycles of violence that bring misery to our lives and ultimately to our world.

Satya

The next *yama* factor is truthfulness, or *satya*, nonlying. The logic behind *satya* as a yogic virtue is that truth is in conformity with reality and that knowing the reality of things is a critical element of spiritual development. It refers, in its most concrete sense, to the idea of lying as intentionally misleading others with words that are not in harmony with the reality of things. In this respect, it is often explained as different from simply sharing a mistaken or misinformed view of things, as it implies obscuring the truth. Leading others astray is harmful to varying degrees and may be motivated by a range of emotions. This obscuring of the truth is harmful to others and an entanglement for the person doing it. A truthful statement conforms to the way that things are, but a lie requires an ongoing process of bending the facts to support its existence. Lying to others chips away at one's inner integrity and may plant itself like a seed in one's consciousness, giving rise to an inability to see oneself honestly. In other words, the outer *satya* of relationships with others might be said to be in relation to an inner *satya*, which is the nature of the relationship with oneself.

It should also be pointed out that the commentarial tradition of yoga emphasizes that *satya* should always be in service of *ahiṃsā*. This means that one should speak carefully and avoid brutal honesty, gossip, and so on, which do more harm than good for others. It also calls for discretion with respect to sharing information about oneself and others that might be used for harmful purposes by others. This is related to the idea that being truthful and being forthcoming or volunteering information are different things. It implies not that criticism of others is inherently wrong but rather that it is important to be mindful of the boundary between constructive criticism and destructive criticism, or even cynicism.

Asteya

Following *satya* is the practice of nonstealing, or *asteya*. The principle of nonharming is evident here, as well, in that stealing is often a cause of pain and suffering for others. Likewise, stealing represents, for yoga, the physical manifestation of greed and ignorance—an overwhelming impulse to obtain objects of desire and an objectified sense of self and other. Stealing may be concrete, in the form of taking physical objects such as money or personal possessions, but also may manifest in the stealing of ideas or in imbalanced emotional relationships that are driven by fear or dependency. Stealing may become socialized or institutionalized in a manner that is virtually invisible, and those who are participating in the stealing may or may not be aware that it is happening. Laws may be unjust. Again, the observance of *yama*, broadly speaking, calls for a mindful attitude toward one's life experiences and actions. Through being mindful, one can unearth the small and large ways in which one takes what is not one's own or participates in a community or culture that is in some way benefiting from harmfully taking from others.

Brahmacarya

Brahmacarya, or sexual restraint, has been discussed above, but there are a number of points worth repeating. The first is that *brahmacarya* is an extension of *ahiṃsā*, which means that the litmus test for the moral nature of the expression of sexuality is whether or not it is harmful to others. It requires introspection into the ways that the expression of sexuality can be coercive and destructive, which may involve overcoming previously unconscious assumptions about sexual relationships and having more explicit communication with partners about sexuality. The Indian tradition offers a range of perspectives on what "right" sexual relationships should look like—some remarkably progressive and others that might be viewed as antiquated relics of a bygone era. What is clear, however, is the spirit of this moral principle, which is that unmindful expressions of sexuality can lead to harm and are at odds with the practice of yoga. In addition to the physical and emotional harm of coercive sexual relationships, the expression of sexuality—due to its emotional intensity—is seen as potentially a source of further entanglement in the world. The power of sexual sentiments makes them ripe for addiction and compulsion. The monastic's commitment to celibacy, for example, might be said to be pragmatic, as a recovery of the time and energy otherwise spent on pursuing sexual activity. It might also be said to be idealistic in that it represents one mode of living free from any attachment and thus is coextensive with the ideal of spiritual liberation. On the other hand, the restraint of harmful sexual behavior in its concrete form may be seen as a precursor to changing former ways of thinking. Though thoughts may be subtler and less concrete than physical action, from the viewpoint of much of Indian philosophy they are just as, if not more, important than their counterparts.

Aparigraha

The last of the five *yama* factors is nongreed, or *aparigraha*. The notion that a *yogin* or *yoginī* should restrain the impulse to obtain worldly objects makes perfect sense in a philosophy in which one is trying to achieve contemplative peace. To the degree that life is dedicated to the pursuit of the accumulation of goods, it is difficult to find the time and energy to practice. It is also clear how the hoarding of resources means that others will have to live with less or completely without. The limitlessness of desire, and of greed, lends itself to a self-propagating cycle of having to have more and never being satisfied with less. One way to fruitfully expand on this is to look at *aparigraha* as meaning "nonaddiction." Obtaining objects of desire makes us feel good, at least temporarily. It is addictive, and it pushes us to more and greater acquisition. Addiction to drugs and alcohol demonstrates how our attachment to an object can cloud our perception, leading to cycles of abuse and profound harm for the user and those around them. Anyone who has struggled with financial debt understands how easily a person can fall into a downward-spiraling cycle that saps one's resources and casts a pall over one's life. Yoga might be thought of in this regard as an approach to overcoming both material and psychic debts, ways of thinking and acting that bind us to misery and lead us into more entanglement. As we struggle to cover the "overhead" of our material and psychic needs, we risk compromising our moral decisions. The positive side of this equation, from a yogic perspective, is that we can become habituated in *aparigraha* such that we become increasingly able to avoid entanglement and to extricate ourselves from the spirit of possessiveness that is at the root of so much of our suffering in this world.

It is also worth noting that a key traditional expression of *aparigraha* is the nonacceptance of gifts. This ties into the idea that a gift contains an implicit exchange of power or influence in which the receiver of the gift is expected to be indebted in some way to the giver. In other words, gift giving might be thought of as a form of spiritual lobbying whereby the giver attempts to establish influence over the receiver. Most of us have some level of experience with the dynamics of gift giving within our families and a sense of how such exchanges affect the emotional and power dynamics between people. These issues often come to the fore when a practitioner develops a popular following and thus draws a greater amount of attention from a range of people and interests.

Mastery of *Yama*

According to the *Yogasūtra* verses that outline what happens when these *yama* factors become established or mastered, habitual practice (*abhyāsa*) of *yama* brings about a certain momentum, an ease and perfection that support and enhance spiritual life. With *ahiṃsā*, the aggression of other beings ceases in the presence of the practitioner—he or she effectively creates an aura of peace in the space around them. Establishment in *satya* leads to a state of "fruitful action," interpreted to mean either that the words of the practitioner make things come to be or that the practitioner's actions bear appropriate fruit, as there is no disparity between intention and deed. The second interpretation is particularly coherent, suggesting that when a person is truly honest with herself and others, she will act in such a way that her deeds will be fruitful in the manner intended. With respect to *asteya*, the text states that "all jewels approach" the person who has achieved mastery, suggesting that either material or spiritual wealth, or both, comes to those who refrain from taking what is not theirs. The established practice of *brahmacarya* is said to result in obtaining a vigor or energy (*vīrya*) that is conducive to spiritual development and the obtaining of yogic powers.

Lastly, mastery of *aparigraha* is said to lead to an insight into the nature of life, the "how" of existence, which emerges when the clouds of craving and greed begin to dissipate. Together, these five powers are said to result from the mastery of the elements of *yama*, demonstrating how the restraint of mundane or worldly activities yields a corresponding spiritual mastery. Like the limbs of yoga themselves, the *yama* factors operate in such a way that the perfection of each *yama* strengthens and helps to perfect the others. The *yama* factors provide fertile ground for the development of the succeeding limbs of yoga, as well as being reflective in important ways of what embodied enlightenment looks like.

3

Niyama

OBSERVANCE

YS II.45 *samādhisiddhirīśvarapraṇidhānāt*

Through dedication to Īśvara, [there is] mastery of *samādhi*.

Overview of *Niyama*

The practice of yogic observance, or *niyama*, is the second limb of the *aṣṭāṅgayoga* series and a logical step forward that builds on the practice of *yama*. The practice of *yama* is oriented principally toward social relationships, with the goal of cultivating a mode of life that limits the destructive harming of oneself and others. *Niyama*, on the other hand, refers principally to the more subtle, and constructive, actions that one takes toward oneself in cultivating the practice of yoga and deepening one's spiritual life. Georg Feuerstein, a contemporary scholar of yoga, has put it in this way: *yama* is what one does when others are looking, and *niyama* is what one does when others are not looking. *Niyama* can be thought of as the private counterpart to the public practice of *yama*. It should be kept in mind, though, that *yama* can refer to inner practices of *ahiṃsā* and the like, and *niyama* likewise has social implications and can be practiced in a communal setting. This basic distinction is nevertheless useful for getting an initial sense of the shift from the public and social sphere toward the private and personal sphere of practice that takes place in moving from *yama* to *niyama*. The idea of progressing from the concrete and expansive toward the more subtle and inward is representative of the progression of the limbs of yoga as a whole. Having established a foundation in a moral mode of living in the world, a practitioner of yoga then turns to cultivating a spiritual discipline that informs and inspires his or her performance of yoga. The factors of *niyama* include purity (*śauca*), contentment (*saṃtoṣa*), self-discipline (*tapas*), self-study (*svādhyāya*), and dedication to the lord (*īśvarapraṇidhāna*).

Śauca

The first element of *niyama* is purity, or *śauca*, which literally means something like "cleanliness." "Purity" would be a less literal translation, but it captures the notion that this foundation of yogic practice implies both physical and spiritual cleanliness, the former in service of the latter. Indian religious traditions, especially Hinduism, have long associated cleanliness with spiritual purity in important ways. This continues to be a highly important part of the ritual life of contemporary Hindu Brahmins (from the term *brāhmaṇa*, often translated as "priest"), for whom daily ritual baths are of great significance. Bathing and personal cleanliness are of significance in the broader scope of Hinduism and are exemplified by public ablutions at religious sites of significance, such as on the steps leading into the Ganges river in Banaras.

Bathing is viewed as a proper precursor to worshipping a deity in one's home or in a temple, in a manner that might be compared with rituals of washing that Muslims and Roman Catholics perform before religious services.

There is a deeper paradigm here, perhaps universal in scope, which is the connection between the purification of the body as a preparation for encountering the spirit and performing religious activities in various traditions. This builds on the more mundane or pragmatic considerations of the connection between physical health and cleanliness (such as washing hands, etc.). *Śauca* is also applied to the diet, what one "takes in"—typically, the prescribed diet of the *yogin* or *yoginī* is of a healthy, light (*sattva*) nature, which is conducive to physical well-being and fruitful spiritual practice. The traditions of *haṭhayoga* include elaborate practices of bodily purification, such as the cleansing of the nostrils with a thread or stream of water. The idea of physical cleansing is complemented by ideas about the cleansing of the internal dimensions of thought and emotion, achieved through working to uproot negative states, such as anger, and cultivating positive ones. One contemporary formulation of the Buddhist path summarizes spiritual practice as involving three things: abstention from harm, doing good, and purifying the mind. These all can be viewed both as steps on the path and as the culmination of the practice of yoga. They help provide a foundation for contemplative practice and are viewed as an enlightened attitude to life in an embodied human form.

The practice of *śauca* can be observed as part of one's larger lifestyle and as a matter of habit. It can also be an object of focus in preparation for practice. Removing clutter from one's home and practice space can provide a tangible spaciousness and openness that is supportive of practice.

Daily bathing would be another key example of how purity can be practiced in everyday life, with attention paid to caring for one's own bodily cleanliness. This might be augmented by washing for more directed activities, such as bathing or showering before practicing yoga postures or meditation. One might also take time in the morning to set one's mental intention for the day—cultivating attitudes of friendliness and kindness, trying to reduce feelings or thoughts of anger, and so forth by meditating on directing loving-kindness (*maitrī*) and compasssion (*karuṇā*) toward oneself and the people in one's life. This might be complemented by focused attempts to mentally prepare for a session of yoga, to "clear the air" in the mind, so to speak, so that practice time can be utilized most fully. It makes sense that one should be mindful of and attentive to the negative attitudes and emotions that one brings to the practice of yoga, so as to lessen their disruptive power.

Saṃtoṣa

The next factor or element of *niyama* is contentment, or *saṃtoṣa*. The notion of contentment is striking in its countercultural force with regard to the dominant attitudes of our time, particularly the affliction of greed. What *saṃtoṣa* calls for, as a practice, is the cultivation of an attitude of contentment with regard to our current situation in life. In other words, it is a conscious cultivation of an attitude that accepts the conditions of the present moment, a striving for balance, or ecology, in one's life. It presupposes the idea that we can recalibrate our inner attitudes so that we are content no matter what our circumstances are and live in a way that is sustainable and supportive of practice. Most of us have experienced the reality of obtaining some lifelong goal or object only to find that it does not offer the satisfaction that we thought it would. This is typically because our appetites have grown larger and more sophisticated, and what would have satisfied us at one point in life will not in another. This is not to say that *saṃtoṣa* is a blind acceptance of the way things are without the motivation to change or improve one's circumstances. In fact, it might be argued that meaningful change begins with acceptance, and contentment for what one has now, even if one is striving for better things. In the practice of yoga *āsana*, for example, many of us have experienced injury due to overaggressive practice, rooted in our impatience and inability to be content with where we are in our practice. There is a type of fine-tuning involved in finding the place where one appreciates where one is at in one's practice, while still pressing forward. The practice of *saṃtoṣa*, which might be likened to counting one's blessings, is an effective tool in modulating one's practice and one's life in such a way as to avoid fruitless overexertion and impatience. The simple life offered by the application of *saṃtoṣa* is one in which a life of fewer things means less stress and more steadiness, where wants and needs are no longer conflated with one another. It is contentment and not complacency, a source of stability in the face of the uncertainty of life. It provides a solid foundation for a sustainable spiritual practice.

Tapas

The practice of *saṃtoṣa* is followed in the *niyama* series by asceticism, or *tapas*. *Tapas* literally means something like "heat."

This is the heat or friction caused by the practice of asceticism (self-denial or self-mortification), a working through of the resistance of conditioning. *Tapas* is pushing the mind and body to their limits for the sake of spiritual discipline. Historically speaking, this was in some cases represented by exposing oneself for prolonged periods of time to the rays of the sun or the heat of a blazing fire. It has also been represented by the practice of intense fasting and other restraints of mind and body. *Tapas* might be considered a forerunner of yoga in that it is an ancient practice of self-discipline that utilizes the human mind and body for spiritual transformation. However, it makes sense to place *tapas* within the framework of *aṣṭāṅgayoga*, with *tapas* representing one aspect of self-discipline among the range of practices that are related systematically under the rubric of yoga. *Tapas* is viewed as having a purifying effect, which lends to the understanding of *tapas* as a preparatory practice with regard to posture and meditation. In the ancient Hindu literature, *tapas* was viewed as potent preparation for ritual and as a source of supernatural powers and abilities with a morally ambiguous character. Hindu literature contains numerous examples of individuals who become powerful through *tapas* and then wield their power in malevolent ways. This again points to the importance of the practice of *yama* as a foundation for practice.

The discipline of *tapas* can be compared fruitfully with contemporary calisthenic and athletic cultures in which vigorous workouts are prized for their physical and psychological benefits. Running, for example, might be thought of as both literally and figuratively creating heat—the intense heat of the body in exertion in the first case and the friction between the discomfort of the body and the mental will to move forward in the second. In some cases, running presses extreme physical boundaries, such as in marathons or ultramarathons. The aerobic and anaerobic intensity of the activity has measurable physiological effects, increasing blood flow, causing mood-altering chemicals to enter the bloodstream, and so forth. Vigorous systems of contemporary yoga, such as the *aṣṭāṅga vinyāsa* system and "flow yoga," or generic *vinyāsa* traditions, might be viewed as incorporating *tapas* within *āsana* practice. The great popularity of hot styles of yoga, such as that of Bikram Choudhury, for example, may well be in part due to the intense catharsis or sense of emotional release provided by the intense heat and perspiration. Likewise, restrictive diets produce not only weight loss but often feelings of control or mastery over one's mental and emotional life. Any of these practices can be taken to the extreme, whether in yogic or other contexts, and can lead to physical or mental harm. Much as is the case with Buddhism, the philosophical traditions of yoga we are discussing place emphasis on the instrumental nature of ascetic practices, and stop short of self-harm. The "middle way" philosophy of Buddhism, for example, hinges upon the idea that neither indulgence nor self-harm is spiritually profitable; one should avoid extremes, pursuing self-discipline that strengthens mind and body and provides suitable conditions for cultivating spiritual insight. However, just as the physical strength and emotional stability provided by athletic conditioning do not necessitate moral behavior on the part of an athlete, ascetic discipline or *tapas* does not make a person moral or spiritual, though it may facilitate moral or spiritual development. B.K.S. Iyengar, a key figure in the formulation of modern yoga, stated that practicing the postures of yoga without the observance of *yama* and *niyama* is nothing but calisthenics, suggesting that having a moral framework is what makes *tapas* a part of *yoga*.

Svādhyāya

The development of self-study, or *svādhyāya*, the fourth of the five *niyama* factors, can be said to have two principal meanings to the modern yoga practitioner, one conventional and one of a more technical nature. In contemporary yoga traditions, *svādhyāya* is primarily understood in terms of its literal meaning, "self-study," and emphasis is placed upon the process of becoming spiritually reflective. This may be further expanded to mean something to the effect of self-education, or dedication to learning about oneself through the study of yoga. In relation to the idea of *tapas* being about pushing one's limits, *svādhyāya* can be understood as coming to find and accept those limits. The more technical meaning of the term, which is coextensive with the conventional meaning in some ways, is something like "self-recitation." This technical meaning comes from the ancient Hindu Vedic tradition, in which the central ritual act of spiritual life was the recitation of religious verses of sacred texts that had been committed to memory. Drawing from this context, *svādhyāya* can be defined as the recitation of the literature of yoga with an emphasis on the memorization and internalization of text. So, for example, one might obtain a text such as the *Yogasūtra* and read it aloud, trying to grasp its meaning. Likewise, one might take up the recitation of other spiritual or religious texts that are inspirational—perhaps Hindu texts such as the *Bhagavadgītā* or Buddhist texts such as the *Dhammapada*, or alternately the Bible, Qur'an, Torah, and so forth. *Svādhyāya* might also involve the performance of *mantra* (incantations or chants, such as OṂ) known as *jāpa*, prayers, and other formulaic expressions of faith and devotion. One point worth emphasizing here is that *svādhyāya*, in this sense, is a combination of performance and study in which both the spirit and the meaning of the text are brought to life.

Īśvarapraṇidhāna

The last of the *niyama* factors is *īśvarapraṇidhāna*, which means something like "dedication to the lord" or "dedication to the master." In the *Yogasūtra*, Īśvara is described as being a person (*puruṣa*) who has never been caught up and bound by the world in the manner that ordinary people have. He is also described as being the possessor of omniscience and as having manifested in the world in order to teach the principles of yoga to humanity over the course of time. Many contemporary commentators refer to Īśvara simply as "God," given his powers and capacities as described in the philosophical literature of yoga, such as omniscience. In the first section of the *Yogasūtra*, *īśvarapraṇidhāna* is discussed as being a potent manner of eliminating obstacles to the development of contemplation (*samādhi*). The primary practice of *īśvarapraṇidhāna* is recitation and contemplation of the mantra OṂ, known as *praṇava*, which is considered the representative sound of Īśvara. This forms a particular type of devotion (*bhakti*), an intense emotive focusing that is said to accelerate spiritual development. One way to conceive of the operation of Īśvara is in the manner of an intense religious commitment. Through transforming one's practice into an act of devotion, emphasis on one's own ego is diminished and the power of religious sentiment fuels enthusiasm for the practice. In the formula of *tapas-svādhyāya-īśvarapraṇidhāna*, Īśvara is accepting what is beyond one's capacities once one's limits have been tested and accepted. Another approach is to view Īśvara as an archetype or model of what the practitioner hopes to become. Īśvara in this respect represents the radical transcendence of worldly affliction and the ability to manifest, or participate, in the world in an enlightened manner, without getting caught up in it. Developing an intense focus on Īśvara in this respect is like developing an intense focus on the state toward which a practitioner of yoga aspires. For those who find the idea of believing in or developing devotion to a deity unacceptable, the cultivation of devotion and attentiveness to a spiritual ideal might be more acceptable. These two possibilities are not mutually exclusive, either, as the person who views Īśvara in literal terms may still value the manner in which he serves as a model for what a *yogin* or *yoginī* aims to become. The recitation of *praṇava*, or OṂ, is joined with contemplation of the nature of Īśvara as radically transcendent, free from the pain and misery of worldly affliction and manifesting in the world for the benefit of living beings. For some, it may be helpful to conceive of Īśvara in personal terms, in the form of an enlightened deity or sage, such as Śiva, Viṣṇu, Devī, Gaṇeśa, or a buddha or bodhisattva figure. Some practitioners of yoga might find it helpful to construct a small shrine with an image (*mūrti*) that can provide focus to the practice of this aspect of yoga.

Mastery of *Niyama*

As is the case with the five *yama* factors, it is said that mastery of the five *niyama* factors leads particular benefits and powers to arise. In the case of purity (*śauca*), a range of benefits are stated, including the development of a degree of detachment toward one's own and others' bodies, the arising of ease in the body and mind, one-pointedness of mind, control of the senses, and fitness for self-knowledge. The mastery of *saṃtoṣa* is said to yield unexcelled happiness, implying that the greatest happiness in life is to be found through cultivating contentment rather than through the process of accumulation. *Tapas* is said to result in the perfection of the body and senses through the destruction of impurities, leading to the attainment of "yoga powers." These powers, according to the commentarial literature, include the development of heightened perceptual abilities and a malleability of one's physical form. The mastery of the practice of *svādhyāya* is said to lead to union with one's desired deity (*iṣṭadevatā*). One way to interpret this is that as one recites a text or mantra with intensity of purpose, the truth of that text becomes transparent—in the case of a mantra, one gains communion with the sacred reality or principle that it represents, such as a deity. Likewise, one might be said to gain communion with the thoughts or mind of the author of a philosophical text and thus gain deep insight into the author's mind and the object of study. Lastly, through *īśvarapraṇidhāna*, it is said that the practitioner of yoga quickly perfects *samādhi*, or meditative contemplation. Devotion or dedication to Īśvara is thus thought of as a sort of shortcut that leads in rapid fashion to the achievement of deep meditative contemplation and ultimately to liberation.

As discussed previously, the elements of *yama* and *niyama* can be seen as precursors to the other limbs of yoga in that they provide a foundation and context for practice. It is clear, however, that they constitute in and of themselves important practices that are instrumental in the process of spiritual development up to the attainment of liberation. Having established the practice of *yama* and *niyama*, we can now take up the successive limbs of yoga, beginning with the practice of posture (*āsana*), the touchstone of many contemporary yoga traditions.

4

Āsana · Prāṇāyāma · Pratyāhāra

POSTURE • BREATH CONTROL • SENSE WITHDRAWAL

YS II.46 *sthirasukham āsanam*
Posture is [characterized by] stability and comfort.

Āsana

The practice of physical posture, or *āsana*, is a fundamental and iconic aspect of contemporary yoga traditions and the aspect that is of greatest visibility within the global dissemination of yoga. This is the case for a number of reasons. One is that posture has a long and important history within yoga traditions, being an aspect of the process of self-control, or "yoking" the body and mind. Another reason is that many contemporary yoga traditions place a significant emphasis on posture, bringing it to the forefront of the practice. The postural dimension of yoga translates effectively across cultural boundaries; it is not as tied up in metaphysical or philosophical concerns; and it links up in important ways with larger global cultures of the body, such as athletics and calisthenics. Many modern proponents of yoga, perhaps most notably B.K.S. Iyengar, helped bring yoga into popular consciousness through highlighting how the most tangible and visible aspect of yoga—*āsana*, or posture—can be a contemplative exercise in itself, and how *āsana* practice can contain a profound degree of subtlety and complexity, producing insight into the body and mind. It is common for proponents of contemporary yoga traditions to see all of the other eight limbs of yoga within *āsana*, or to argue that although *āsana* is the third limb in the *aṣṭāṅgayoga* series, it is in fact the limb that is to be practiced first. Posture has become a touchstone for the practice of modern yoga, and it is entirely appropriate, if not necessary, for yoga to be contextualized in such a way that makes it relevant to its contemporary audience. However, most practitioners come to recognize quickly that *āsana* is but one aspect of the larger picture of the practice of yoga.

Āsana literally means "seat," coming from the Sanskrit verbal root √*ās*, "to sit," being similar to the relationship between the words "seat" and "sit" in the English language. In the *Yogasūtra*, the practice of *āsana* is mentioned only briefly. Patañjali mentions *āsana* in three verses of the *Yogasūtra* (YS II.46–48). It is quite possible that Patañjali is just discussing *āsana* in the form of seated postures that would be suitable for the practice of meditation. However, the principles that Patañjali articulates are applicable more widely to a range of yogic postures, to the *aṣṭāṅgayoga* system as a whole, and to subsequent systems of yoga. The primary commentator on the *Yogasūtra*, Vyāsa, lists a total of eleven postures. These are principally postures that occur on the ground, including the lotus posture (*padmāsana*) and staff pose (*daṇḍāsana*). Later *haṭhayoga*, or medieval traditions, added significantly to the number of poses included in the rubric of yoga, with the number of *āsana* variations discussed ranging from eighty-four to eighty-four thousand. In *haṭhayoga*, as well as in the yoga philosophy we have been discussing, *āsana* appears largely as a practice done on the ground, and often in support of the practices of *prāṇāyāma* or meditation (*dhyāna*). In modern yoga traditions, the vocabulary of poses has grown significantly, with a much greater emphasis on the use of standing postures and on the idea of linking postures together in an organized or systematic fashion as a "flow."

The practice of *āsana* as a member of the *aṣṭāṅgayoga* system hinges upon the idea that the perfection of posture leads to a state of being resistant or impervious to the stresses of the "pairs of opposites," or the extremes that nature throws at us. The first *Yogasūtra* verse on *āsana* simply defines it as being characterized by stability (*sthira*) and ease or comfort (*sukha*), an integration of complementary principles. This makes sense with respect to the idea that *āsana* is a precursor to *prāṇāyāma* and meditation, in which a practitioner would presumably sit for a long period of time. This requires stability (or effort), which holds the body upright, and a degree of ease that prevents the posture from becoming too stiff or uncomfortable and thus distracting. This can, and has been, extended more broadly to talk about a larger range of postures within modern and contemporary yoga traditions. The practice of *āsana*, the hallmark of many modern yoga traditions, is often characterized as a balance of these two factors.

The second verse on *āsana* (YS II.47) can also be applied to a range of standing postures, as well as to static sitting postures. It states, according to most authorities, that *āsana* is established as such by means of the "relaxation of effort" and "meditation on the infinite." This is often interpreted to mean that mastery of yoga postures results from the combination of relaxing into a posture and directing the mind toward the infinite, as a sense of either directing the mind endlessly in one direction or concentrating upon the divine. Another translation, which is perhaps not as straightforward, would be something to the effect of "by the endless unification of effort and relaxation." This second translation is compelling in that it captures, as in the first verse, the idea of bringing stability and ease together in a continuous fashion.

The third verse (YS II.48) states that mastery of *āsana* yields a state of being free from the "assault of the opposites," such as hot and cold, a perfection of the practice akin to those of *yama* and *niyama*. This is intuitively coherent for anyone who has practiced *āsana* in a significant way—cultivating the ability to sit or stand with stability in a posture requires stamina, mental discipline, and a tolerance for stress, qualities that typically extend into one's larger life. Disturbance is understood as the disequilibrium of duality, which ceases in the integration of complementary forces. This thread, which runs clearly through the practice of *āsana* and anchors it as a spiritual practice, is the effort-ease dynamic, a permutation of the pair of practice (*abhyāsa*) and detachment (*vairāgya*) that undergirds yoga practice. This is one way in which yoga *āsana* might be seen to represent foundational principles of yoga. Many of us with *āsana* practices can identify with the experience of finding the "sweet spot" in an *āsana*, where we have managed to fine-tune the level of effort and ease in a posture so that it becomes energetically fulfilling and has a calming and focusing effect upon the mind. This is true whether the practice of posture is viewed as a preliminary practice or as an end in itself. It also points to the idea that the factors of *aṣṭāṅgayoga* are linked together by the overarching principles of spiritual practice and liberation.

Despite the differing presentations of the nature and role of *āsana* in the variations of the yoga tradition, the principles articulated in yoga philosophy apply across the spectrum in a number of ways. *Āsana* serves in all cases to awaken the mind and intelligence to progressively more subtle internal perceptions and external factors and effects. Attention to the details of mental, emotional, and physical-structural aspects of *āsana* are complemented by the recognition of the ways in which one's life in the world—such as sleeping, eating, and working—affect one's practice. This internal and external "pattern watching" mirrors the activity of the other limbs of yoga, as does the practice of gracefully approximating a pose in order to grow into a more complete expression of it. It also reveals the inner dynamisms of the body, the sun and moon forces—such as bending forward and backward or inhaling and exhaling—that structurally and energetically complement and counterbalance each other.

Yoga often requires that one choose the harder course among various options in order to channel thoughts and actions toward greater effectiveness and efficiency. This type of behavior modification requires disciplined decision making that forgoes instant gratification for a greater goal. The mastery of the "survival wiring" of the human organism through *āsana* practice allows a practitioner to manage the experiences of fear, discomfort, and pain at the boundaries of one's limits. This requires an inner strength, and *āsana* might be viewed as akin to, or as a mode of, *tapas*, which is a method of training one's will to tolerate the strain of difficult choices and to negotiate one's present mode of living with the lofty ideals of *yama* and *niyama*.

Prāṇāyāma

Along with *āsana*, *prāṇāyāma* is one of the most common and recognizable practices in contemporary yoga. Many contemporary yoga traditions embrace the modern yoga form of *vinyāsa*, in which *āsana* is performed in concert with breath control. The common sun salutation, or *sūrya-namaskāra*, exemplifies this conception—upward and backward stretching are associated with inhalation; forward bending, with exhalation; and so forth. A key example of a *prāṇāyāma* utilized in *āsana* practice is *ujjāyī prāṇāyāma*, the "victorious breath control," a *haṭhayoga* technique that is often integrated into *vinyāsa* practice, bringing intensity and control to the breath-movement link. The legacy of the medieval *haṭhayoga* traditions thus carries forward into the present through the continuation of a range of *prāṇāyāma* forms that are discussed in the *Haṭhayogapradīpikā* and other texts. Even in contexts where formal *prāṇāyāma* is not practiced as part of yoga, some aspect of breath awareness or control is typically taught as facilitating strength, stamina, and flexibility in static poses. According to K. Pattabhi Jois, one of the key figures in the development of modern yoga traditions, performing *āsana* without proper *prāṇāyāma* technique is simply physical exercise. Developing attention to, or mindfulness of, the breathing process may well be one of the hallmarks of contemporary yoga traditions, even in their most stripped-down forms. One of the lessons of modern yoga is that *āsana* practice requires a heightened consciousness of the breathing process. Developing strength, stamina, and flexibility in *āsana* practice often requires the deepening of the breath and the development of increasingly subtle control over the movements of body and breath. Both *āsana* and *prāṇāyāma* could thus be said to override the "survival wiring" of the human body, establishing volitional control over aspects of one's embodiment that are otherwise set within certain given parameters and autonomous in operation.

As with *āsana*, the discussion of *prāṇāyāma* is given a limited number of verses in the *Yogasūtra*—a total of five. The first verse simply defines *prāṇāyāma* as the stopping of the movement of the inhalation and exhalation of breath. In other words, the basic principle of *prāṇāyāma* is the controlling of the movement of inhalation and exhalation. The second verse on *prāṇāyāma* provides a more detailed analysis of this process of control, noting that it can be broken down into "external," "internal," and "suppressed," and observed in terms of place, time, and number. The drawing of breath becomes increasingly long and subtle. The key ideas here involve the notions of what are referred to as *recaka*, *pūraka*, and *kumbhaka* in *haṭhayoga* and modern yoga traditions: namely, exhalation, inhalation, and retention. One well-known example is the 1:4:2 sequence of timing with respect to inhalation, retention, and exhalation, in which the proportionate length of the count of each part follows the formula. One might perform a particular number of repetitions or number of sets of the sequence. Some commentators interpret the second verse as referring specifically to retention and its various forms, which are of particular import in many of the *prāṇāyāma* systems. Whether this is the case or not, what is clear is that great value is placed on bringing systematic regulation to the processes of breathing, specifically these three stages of breath.

The third verse on *prāṇāyāma* in the *Yogasūtra* speaks of a very subtle form, the culmination of the previous practices, which is said to be distinct from either internal or external conditions. This form of *prāṇāyāma* is similar, if not identical, to what is referred to as *kevala kumbhaka* in the *haṭhayoga* traditions, a spontaneous retention of the breath that is independent of either exhalation or inhalation. *Prāṇāyāma* leads progressively to a more subtle movement of breath, which reaches perfection in the form of *kevala kumbhaka*, the ability to spontaneously make one's breathing profoundly subtle, if not restrained completely. This may imply, again, a "graceful approximation" strategy whereby the more basic forms of *prāṇāyāma* give way to a more complete form, in a manner analogous to the way that an imperfect *āsana* is mastered when the external form of the posture gives way as the internal form reveals itself spontaneously and with ease.

Following the larger pattern we have seen with respect to the limbs of yoga, Patañjali dedicates two verses to describing the effects of perfecting breath control in this manner. The first verse states that there is the destruction of the "covering of the light," which is typically interpreted to mean that *prāṇāyāma* has a purifying force on the mind, uncovering its natural radiance. The principal commentaries state that the "residue" of our actions (*karma*) in life obscures the light of the intellect or knowledge, and *prāṇāyāma* clears that residue, or mental fog, away. Vyāsa states that in this regard, *prāṇāyāma* can be thought of as the foremost type of *tapas*, or purifying act of self-discipline, one that helps purify and clarify the mind itself. The final verse on *prāṇāyāma* points to the implications of such purification: the mind is said to become fit for the practice of *dhāraṇā*, the fixation or concentration of the mind, the first "internal limb" of yoga. In this regard, *prāṇāyāma* might be viewed as the foundation for the development of meditation, a viewpoint that is echoed in the texts of *haṭhayoga*, in which the attainment of perfection in *prāṇāyāma* is said to perfect *haṭhayoga* and lead to the development of deep meditative absorption or contemplation, referred to as the "royal yoga" (*rājayoga*). One way to interpret this physiologically would be to see *prāṇāyāma* as regulating the impulses of the nervous system so as to effectively force the system into a state of focused receptivity.

It could be drawn from these assertions that *prāṇāyāma* as a discipline progressively works to bring clarity to the mind through purifying it of the aftereffects of one's actions (*karma*), leading toward a state where the mind's natural propensity to become concentrated becomes active. Without doubt, innumerable contemporary yoga practitioners could testify to the power of breath awareness, or *prāṇāyāma*, in bringing about a focused and concentrated mental state. For many contemporary traditions of yoga, and especially in *vinyāsa*-based traditions, the breath is the glue that holds practice together, bringing unity and coherence to a variety of postures and practices and bridging the gap between the external and internal limbs. Though the pursuit of more sophisticated and complex types of *prāṇāyāma* may be limited to the highly motivated and often more experienced practitioners of yoga, even the most elementary forms of breath awareness and breath control embody the principles of the practice in concrete ways.

Pratyāhāra

The fifth limb of yoga, *pratyāhāra*, receives limited discussion in the *Yogasūtra* text and commentaries. It is described as a process of withdrawal, in which the senses turn away from their objects and become like, or follow, the mind because they are no longer dependent on their objects of perception. It is said that *pratyāhāra* leads to the highest control of the senses or sense organs. The commentarial literature on this verse emphasizes the idea that the process of disciplining the mind naturally causes or includes the disciplining of the senses. It might be best thought of as a practice that is at the transition between *prāṇāyāma* and the development of the meditative process. *Prāṇāyāma* makes the mind "fit" for meditation, and *pratyāhāra* is the effort to draw away from the world of the senses and into the world of the mind.

Contemporary practitioners of yoga *āsana* and meditation will undoubtedly be familiar with *pratyāhāra* to some extent. The foremost example would be the self-conscious attempt to draw one's awareness back to posture or meditation when it is drawn outward by sensory stimuli or into thought. This can be enhanced to some degree through practicing in an environment in which distractions are limited. However, it is impossible to completely avoid distraction, and so an ability to consciously draw awareness back to the body or mind is necessary. Most contemporary *āsana* and meditation practitioners have had the experience of reaching a settled state of practice where the outer world fades away and the immediate object of attention becomes more prominent. Most of us have had experiences of times or particular days when it seemed impossible to keep our attention focused, and other times or days when focus seemed to happen automatically. The principle of yoga practice applied to this situation yields an intuitive, but important, point: sense control is a matter of habit, and the more it is practiced, the more it will be established and regular.

The principle of gaze (*dṛṣṭi*) as an augment to *āsana* practice might be viewed as a way that *pratyāhāra* has been integrated into postural practice. A practice in which each posture has an associated gazing point reins in the focus of *āsana* practice, drawing attention away from the background around the practitioner and into the immediate sphere of practice. Again, those of us who have practiced *āsana* with *dṛṣṭi* will quickly admit that it is not always easy to keep continuously drawing awareness back to our practice and toward the point of focus. However, with regular and committed rehearsal, it can become almost effortless at times. The idea of *dṛṣṭi* also ties in with the idea that *pratyāhāra* is a natural consequence of mental focus; the attention one pays to one's *dṛṣṭi*, such as the tip of the nose or the navel, draws awareness away from the greater environment and concentrates it within the immediate region of practice. Meditation practitioners will also likely identify with the struggle to return attention from sensory or mental distraction and develop the habit of remaining in proximity to the object or field of meditative attention. Techniques such as drawing the limbs into the body and either closing the eyes (if visually distracted) or slightly opening them (if easily falling into imaginative activity or thought) can thus assist in the "introversion" process of meditation.

Gateway to the "Inner Limbs" of Yoga

Pratyāhāra, the fifth limb of *aṣṭāṅgayoga*, is the final external limb of yoga. The domain of the first five limbs begins with the relationship one has with others in the social world and ends with the withdrawal of the senses from their worldly objects. The inner limbs of *dhāraṇā*, *dhyāna*, and *samādhi* are all within the domain of the mind (*citta*). As we have seen with the outer factors of *yama*, *niyama*, *āsana*, *prāṇāyāma*, and *pratyāhāra*, the perfection of the inner factors of *dhāraṇā*, *dhyāna*, and *samādhi* yield particular types of powers and abilities that are of great utility and benefit from the viewpoint of the yoga philosophy. We will turn to these in the next chapter.

5

Dhāraṇā · Dhyāna · Samādhi

CONCENTRATION • MEDITATION • CONTEMPLATION

YS III.4 *trayam ekatra saṃyamaḥ*

The three [*dhāraṇā*, *dhyāna*, and *samādhi*] as one is [yogic] mastery.

The Internal Limbs of Yoga

The final three limbs in the *aṣṭāṅgayoga* system are concentration, or *dhāraṇā*; meditation, or *dhyāna*; and contemplation, or *samādhi*. The three form a coherent unit as the three internal (*antar*) limbs of yoga. Almost half of the verses of the *Yogasūtra* are dedicated to discussing the contemplative processes of the internal limbs of yoga and the results they yield in terms of power and liberation. Early in the third section of the *Yogasūtra*, Patañjali discusses these three limbs as a unit, forming what is called yogic mastery (*saṃyama*), which yields the "light of wisdom" (*prajñā-āloka*). The development of deep meditative contemplation is said to yield insight into whatever the *yogin* or *yoginī* chooses to meditate upon. This insight is portrayed as the source of a range of supernormal powers and capacities within the world and as the gateway to the discernment of the true nature of the self and of the world, leading to spiritual liberation, which is termed "separation" (*kaivalya*). The formulation of these three limbs presents a vision of the profound power of a mind that has been trained to apply itself intensely to an object and abandon all distraction, embodying the foundational dynamic between practice (*abhyāsa*) and dispassion (*vairāgya*) in yoga. Like many smaller streams coming together to make a great and powerful river, the process of meditation brings together the energy of the scattered mind into a focused stream of attention. *Samādhi* is the culmination of the limbs of yoga and is said to bring about the perfection and fulfillment of the others. However, like all of the limbs of yoga, it is a practice dedicated to transformation, and in the state of liberation it is said to become unnecessary. Like a raft that has fulfilled the purpose of crossing a stream, it is abandoned because it is no longer necessary.

Dhāraṇā

Only one verse of the *Yogasūtra* is dedicated to *dhāraṇā*, indicating its preliminary place in the development of yogic mastery. *Dhāraṇā* is defined literally as the "binding of the mind to a place." It is the initial moment of concentration or fixation of the mind in meditation, the willful engagement with an object of meditation. It could also be thought of as the application of the mind to an object, a choosing to single out some aspect of the world for definitive focus. Concentration is the hallmark of meditation and relies upon both the habituation of fixing the mind on an object and the abandoning of distractions. Objects include, for example, the mantra OṂ or the movement of the breath; the chief commentator on the *Yogasūtra* also mentions it can be places such as the navel, the heart, the top of the head, the tip of the nose, or a physical object in the world. Having chosen an object, such as the mantra OṂ or the movement of the breath, the mind is placed upon or focused on that object distinctly and with attentive energy. The untrained mind, habituated to fluctuate, will soon draw the attention away to other objects, such as memories, sensory stimuli, or thoughts about the past or future. Having noticed such distraction, the meditator returns the mind to its original object and attempts to establish concentration once again. This process is quite simple in theory but requires persistent and determined effort to carry out. The untrained mind is unruly, and it can be difficult not to get frustrated by the propensity of the mind to become distracted, sometimes for long periods of time. However, with patience and discipline, the mind is habituated to staying on an object, and it becomes considerably easier to sustain concentration, leading to the development of meditation (*dhyāna*). The dynamic forces of *abhyāsa* and *vairāgya* are present in the form of bringing additional energy or tension to concentration, if necessary, or easing up and settling down on an object when the mind is too rigid. Fine-tuning the level of energy and exertion is key to avoid having attention be so lax as to lose the object to mental dullness, or so tight that the mind scatters excitedly to other things. Both classical and contemporary sources on Buddhist meditation put great emphasis on the need to modulate or adjust the intensity of concentration, especially of tension and relaxation, to achieve balance. With practice, the mind becomes unified on the object and achieves a "one-pointed" (*ekāgratā*) state.

Dhyāna

Dhyāna is a term that is used in many contexts to refer to the larger practice or process of meditation. In the context of *aṣṭāṅgayoga* it also has a more technical meaning, which builds upon the practice of *dhāraṇā*. The definition of *dhyāna* in this context is "an extension of the unity of the basis." What this means is that *dhyāna* is the stretching out, or extension of, the unification of the mind on an object that is characteristic of *dhāraṇā*. *Dhāraṇā* is characterized by momentary concentration on an object, and *dhyāna* is the extension of that concentration into a flowing process. *Dhyāna* is the perfection of the process of habituation in *dhāraṇā*—rather than having moments of concentration, now the process becomes continuous and sustained, leading to a deeper and more peaceful state of meditation. This represents a greater level of subtlety being brought to the adjustments in intensity and relaxation in one's concentration. In *dhyāna*, the continuity of fixation on the object is not lost for successively longer periods of time, and so concentration becomes more subtle and engrossing. The habit-energy of concentration has now borne fruit in the form of continuity of attention on the object of one's choosing. In some Buddhist sources, it is emphasized that just as one has to recognize the more concrete reality of distraction in losing the object completely in *dhāraṇā*, in *dhyāna* it is important to recognize the subtle distractions of a dull mind or an excited one and adjust intensity to counter these influences, lest they precipitate full-blown distraction. This requires more subtle skill and mindfulness, which take experience in practice to develop. However, just as one can develop an ability over time to negotiate the tension-relaxation dynamic of practicing an *āsana*, it is a matter of consistent application that leads to negotiating the similar principles in meditation. Likewise, one might expect that the attainment of meditative focus in *āsana* would predispose a person to accelerated mastery of *dhyāna* and that the experienced practitioner of *dhyāna* would quickly grasp the fine-tuning of *āsana* as well. In both *āsana* and *dhyāna*, the ability to respond to and anticipate disequilibrium through a potentially infinite range of compensatory movements is at the basis of achieving a spontaneous and dynamic mastery.

Samādhi

The perfection of *dhyāna* leads to the final limb of yoga, *samādhi*. The term *samādhi* itself means something akin to "contemplation." It is described in the *Yogasūtra* as being a state in which an object of meditation shines forth as if in a state of emptiness, due to the cessation of any thought or stimulus that would draw the mind away from the object. Concentration has become perfected in *samādhi*, and there is a dawning of insight into the nature of the object that is meditated upon—a deep, penetrating awareness that unlocks the mystery of things and that yields, potentially, both power and liberation. One way of analyzing this is to see the development of *samādhi* as a perfecting of the qualities of *dhāraṇā* and *dhyāna* to such an extent that there is an effortless contemplation of the object of concentration. The point of perfect balance between effort and relaxation has been achieved, and so the mind locks on to an object without wavering or exhausting itself. Buddhist sources use a term that is often translated as "pliancy" to express the manner in which the formerly inflexible mind can now be employed fruitfully however the practitioner wills. As discussed earlier, in this aspect, yoga can be seen as an antidote to the struggle for integrity in life and for developing the discipline to rein in one's physical and mental abilities in the service of spiritual development. It is also worth mentioning that these states of meditation are viewed as being increasingly peaceful or blissful. As the fluctuations of the mind settle down and the scattered energies and emotions are brought together and away from distraction, the practitioner experiences states of peace and intense bliss due to being free of the burden of afflicted emotions. Ultimately, it is understood that *samādhi* can facilitate bringing all mental fluctuations to a standstill, to a point of such perfect calm that the true nature of the self and world is understood and spiritual liberation is experienced. Moments of peace are said to give way to a continuous experience of serenity in the face of the flux of life.

Samādhi is typically divided into two forms, *saṃprajñāta* and *asaṃprajñāta*, meaning something to the effect of cognitive and noncognitive *samādhi*. The former is further characterized by four components: application (*vitarka*), consideration (*vicāra*), bliss (*ānanda*), and I-am-ness (*asmitā*). These four factors are coherent with regard to the processes of an object-oriented *samādhi* in that they involve applying and sustaining thought on an object, they result in bliss, and they are centered in the egoic identity of the practitioner. The second type of *samādhi* is characterized by the absence of an object and is therefore sometimes referred to as unconscious *samādhi*. However, it is better referred to as noncognitive, because it is a suppression not of consciousness or awareness but of mental activity that is distinct from consciousness. The suppression of mental activity leads to an experience of consciousness that is not confused with the movements of mind. It manifests as the "cloud-bearing-*samādhi*" (*dharmamegha-samādhi*), where the power of concentration overpowers the habit energies of the mind, precipitating a profound spiritual transformation. As this process reaches its zenith, it is said that the "fuel" of mental fluctuations is expended, and there is an end to the experience of any mental or physical affliction by the practitioner, who then rests in primordial unobstructed awareness. Having brought the practice of *samādhi* to its completion, there is nothing more to be accomplished, as the eight limbs have served their purpose. The power of consciousness dawns and there is an experience of profound freedom. However, this is not to say that liberation is necessarily a state of final removal from the world or that there is no longer a purpose to the life of the *yogin* or *yoginī*. Rather, it is to say that the spiritual path of the eight limbs has a completion, and a door opens to a transformed mode of existence in the world, a new beginning.

Though this may all seem quite complicated and technical, it should be noted that the progression of states of *samādhi* discussed here is viewed as a natural progression. In other words, disciplined practice will, in principle, yield the succession of states of *samādhi*, and elaborate technical knowledge is not necessary. Specialized information can be thought of as a sort of useful "road map" through these subtle states of mind. Like all of the limbs of yoga, meditation becomes perfected through disciplined and consistent practice. The foundation for most meditators is a sitting meditation practice, often complemented by walking meditation. Alternating the two has the benefit of easing the strain of protracted sitting periods. Walking meditation is also of benefit to individuals who have physical difficulty sitting for long periods of time.

Most traditional sources encourage setting up a meditation practice in an area that is safe and peaceful. For sitting meditation, a dedicated space is ideal.

It should be remembered that the discipline of yoga is largely about cultivating the force of habit in service of practice. It is important to try to establish a regular time and place to perform meditation. The goal is to habituate oneself so thoroughly that the moment one arrives at the meditation space or place, the mind is inclined to become quiet and concentrated. Although a yoga *āsana* like lotus pose (*padmāsana*) or half lotus is desirable, given the stability it provides to the body, keeping the spine upright and sitting in a simple cross-legged position or even in a chair is acceptable for the sake of comfort. The spine is drawn upright into a comfortable position and the chin is slightly dropped. The tongue rests at the base of the top row of teeth, and the eyes are either closed or slightly open. The meditator then directs attention to a meditation object such as the mantra OṂ or the movement of the breath in and out of the nostrils. When the mind loses the object because of either dullness of mind or scattering to external objects, it is brought back again. This simple process is repeated indefinitely until the mind begins to habituate to concentrating on the given object. Over time, the tendency of the mind to waver will diminish, and thought will become calm and less disturbing.

Many beginning meditators mistakenly believe that meditation is about trying to stop thought, and therefore they spend many hours frustrated by the fact that they can't seem to suppress their own thinking. The point is not to stop thought but rather to mindfully notice distractions, including thought, and return to the object of meditation. If that is done consistently, the mind will naturally quiet down on its own. As the process matures, it becomes easier both to begin and to stay in a meditative state; the mind becomes calm, and one experiences peace and bliss. As *dhāraṇā*, *dhyāna*, and *samādhi* become fully established, the power of concentration dawns, providing confidence in the process and a sense of the potential for transformation that meditation has to offer. According to Buddhist sources, as one enters into an established state of *samādhi*, there is an experience of great bliss, ease, and focus in the mind, one that transcends the limits of one's previous experience of the mind and embodiment. The concentrated mind, honed through meditation, bears insight into whatever it contemplates.

Most practitioners of meditation will find that it is only a short amount of time before their meditation practice starts to transform their everyday life. This is similar to the way in which many people find a yoga *āsana* practice has an unexpected degree of impact on life "off the mat." The peace, tranquillity, and concentration of the dedicated meditation session extend into the activities one performs in daily life. Buddhist sources comment on the profound sense of ease that emanates from meditation practice into daily life, such that one feels one could "walk through walls." As the mind becomes calmer, the abrupt and dramatic fluctuations of the mind are reined in, leading to a high degree of mental and emotional stability. These factors naturally lead to changes in thought and behavior and to a degree of equanimity in the midst of life's ceaseless change. As discussed earlier, as the mind becomes more stable and focused, it becomes significantly easier to practice the other limbs of yoga, which in turn have a reinforcing effect on meditation—the limbs being thus both sequentially and simultaneously practiced. This process builds momentum in one's practice, which becomes easier to sustain and more fruitful. Ordinary life situations and experiences become opportunities for developing concentration, through bringing mindfulness and concentration to bear on them. One may use the breath or a mantra, for example, as a means of obtaining mental stability, tranquillity, and focus in the midst of daily life activities, whether they are pleasant or painful. One may cultivate the ability to look deeply at one's experiences in life, both painful and pleasant, with equanimity. Time on the mat becomes a resource for bringing a depth element to one's whole life rather than serving as a temporary escape. Seeing how yoga transforms one's life becomes a powerful source of motivation to deepen and expand one's practice.

Yoga Powers

From the viewpoint of the yoga philosophy, the transformation of the practitioner of yoga who masters meditation takes on grand proportions. Yogic mastery (*saṃyama*), as discussed above, is viewed as a gateway to worldly power, as well as to liberation. Nearly one-fourth of the *Yogasūtra* is dedicated to describing the range of powers and abilities that are at the disposal of the *yogin* or *yoginī* who has achieved *saṃyama*. These are typically referred to using terms meaning "accomplishment" (*siddhi*) and "power" (*vibhūti*). Gerald Larson, one of the foremost contemporary scholars of the *Yogasūtra*, has noted that there are two primary categories of yoga accomplishments: those of "knowledges" and those of "powers." The first category includes such special modes of knowledge as knowing the past and the future, understanding the sounds made by all beings, reading minds, and knowing the structure of the earth and the body. The second category includes such powers as the ability to become invisible, to have the strength of an elephant, to possess others' bodies, to project oneself out of the body, and to possess heightened sensory powers. One of the most famous examples of such powers is the list of the so-called eight accomplishments, which includes supernormal powers of minification, lightness, magnification, obtaining, willfulness, pervasion, lordship, and mastery of desire. According to Patañjali, a practitioner of yoga who has mastered *saṃyama* becomes virtually omniscient and omnipotent. The sheer amount of attention paid to *siddhi* and *vibhūti* in the yoga philosophy lends to the understanding that these concepts have an important role to play in the development of yoga, whether they are understood as literal descriptions of spiritual attainments or as metaphors for more mundane or worldly accomplishments.

These powers are understood to require careful handling by the practicing *yogin* or *yoginī*. The powers are described as perfections of worldly agency potentially opposed to the development of deeper stages of *samādhi*. The yoga philosophy also discusses the temptations of spiritual success that are said to come as a practitioner gains proficiency. The *Yogasūtra* and its commentaries describe heavenly beings approaching an accomplished practitioner of yoga and encouraging the enjoyment of promises of heaven—such as an indestructible body, heavenly chariots, supernormal powers of vision, divine potions, and beautiful and seductive beings that offer delight in various forms. Patañjali admonishes the practitioner of yoga to remember that taking pride in yogic accomplishment and stopping to enjoy the fruits of one's practice is to risk falling back into pain and misery. This is undoubtedly a cautionary tale about power, one that can be applied not only to the practice of yoga but also to the worlds of politics, sports, celebrity, and so forth. Those who devote themselves to powerful self-discipline might well obtain power and status in the world—but with that power and status comes the possibility of disruption, of falling from the heights. This is one way in which *yama* is a necessary foundation for the development of the later limbs.

Yama shields a practitioner from the dangerous excesses that are possible when self-discipline becomes fruitful. The *yogin* or *yoginī* who has a solid foundation in *yama* will not be as easily swayed by the temptation to use his or her emerging power in ways that lack integrity. To achieve spiritual liberation, the practitioner has to be prepared to give up even the ultimate powers of omniscience and omnipotence, choosing to develop insight into the nature of the world and the self over the exercise of power in the world. Indian literature is filled with stories of practitioners of asceticism and yoga who become extraordinarily powerful through their spiritual discipline and then use that power for malevolent purposes involving power, sex, and wealth. The contemporary yoga scholar David Gordon White refers to them as "sinister *yogīs*." From the perspective of the yoga philosophy, the pursuit of the *siddhi* or *vibhūti* powers for the sake of worldly gain is a waste of one's resources and will lead to future calamity and pain. On the other hand, some commentators on yoga believe that there is a possibility that a yoga practitioner who has gained liberation can utilize such powers for the benefit of others. This perspective is found in certain Buddhist traditions, where enlightened beings such as buddhas and bodhisattvas are portrayed as utilizing various yogic powers for the sake of the well-being of others.

From this viewpoint, yoga powers are to be utilized only out of compassion and not for the sake of satisfying one's own ego-driven aspirations.

One way to look at *siddhi* and *vibhūti* in a more positive light is to view them as signposts in yogic development, indicators of progressive levels of meditative mastery. From this perspective, the manifestation of various supernormal abilities allows a practitioner to identify that they have crossed a threshold in the development of meditation. These could manifest in terms of inner visions or experiences, or as tangible skills or abilities that apply to one's embodied life in the world. Most of us who have practiced yoga at some point have been inspired by the virtuosity or mastery of our teachers, who have demonstrated skill and knowledge that impress upon us their true embodiment of the yoga practice in important ways. Likewise, many of us have experienced at times a sense of mental or physical transformation that gives us a heightened confidence in our abilities to master our world. Often this perspective springs from our experience of overcoming physical or mental limitations, or from experiencing a degree of power or control over some aspect of our embodiment that we did not think was possible before. This is one of the sources of inspiration in the practice of yoga, the sense of accomplishment that transforms our understanding of ourselves.

However, it is important to note that skill and mastery, from the perspective of the yoga philosophy, do not necessarily mean that one has gained enlightenment or liberation. Self-mastery is consistent with the yoga philosophy and facilitates the process of spiritual self-transformation. This is a subtle distinction, but it is very important. From the perspective of the yoga philosophy, self-discipline and self-mastery are to be celebrated to the degree that they reflect the values of *yama* and of spiritual liberation. There are many individuals who have achieved a high degree of mastery of some aspect of yoga but live lives that are profoundly at odds with the principles of *yama* and the ideal of spiritual liberation (*kaivalya*). Likewise, it is possible to mistakenly convince oneself that the outer trappings of one's skill in some aspect of yoga reflect a deeper spiritual realization. In both cases, a certain amount of critical attitude is required: virtuosity or mastery does not necessarily mean a person has good intentions or is spiritually liberated or enlightened.

This point can be further illustrated by examining the various sources of yoga powers or spiritual accomplishment (*siddhi*) mentioned in the *Yogasūtra*. Patañjali states that spiritual accomplishments can be obtained through five sources: birth (*janma*), herbs (*auṣadhi*), incantation (*mantra*), asceticism (*tapas*), and contemplation (*samādhi*). In other words, the types of magical accomplishment mentioned by Patañjali can be secured by means other than the practice of *samādhi*. This is important to take note of, as it clarifies that the attainment of such powers is not essential or unique to the practice of *aṣṭāṅgayoga*. It also implies that these powers have an ambivalent status with respect to moral and spiritual development. In addition to *samādhi*, permutations of two of the sources given are also found within the *aṣṭāṅgayoga* system itself. Incantation (*mantra*) can be said to be an important part of the practices of *svādhyāya* and of *īśvarapraṇidhāna*. *Tapas* is found as an element of *niyama*, and the practice of *prāṇāyāma* is discussed in the commentarial literature as an ideal form of *tapas*. It should be noted, however, that both *mantra* and *tapas* have been applied in extensive ways in Indian traditions that are not formally connected to the practice of yoga.

In other words, *mantra* and *tapas* have been and continue to be practiced outside the sphere of yoga. Likewise, yoga has a complex historical relationship with the use of herbs (*auṣadhi*), especially the notion of using magical or alchemical "potions" for the purpose of obtaining power and self-transformation. With respect to the notion of birth (*janma*), the suggestion is that certain individuals are born with special powers and abilities that are the result of actions—such as the practice of yoga—in a former life. This is consistent with an overarching Indian conception that current life conditions are the effect of former actions in this life and previous lives. It suggests that certain powers or abilities may result from the fruition or ripening of *karma* from the past rather than from practices one is performing in the present.

Much of this makes intuitive sense if we apply these principles to conceptions of self-mastery that are found in our contemporary life. The idea of birth as constitutive of special powers and abilities is evident with respect to our ideas about intellectual and physical capacity. In many of our contemporary communities, there is great emphasis on the idea that the structure and character of the body and mind at birth is highly determinative of a person's future potential. The structure of the physical body and particular mental characteristics may connect with particular types of artistic, athletic, and intellectual activities as a person grows older. However, to view a child with particular abilities or characteristics as inherently "better" or of greater value than another is clearly a highly problematic moral viewpoint for many reasons. Just as one can make the mistake of viewing an adept at yoga as being an inherently moral or spiritual person, so too can we make the mistake of believing that a person gifted with particular physical or mental talents that are rewarded in society is inherently of value in some way that others are not.

As analogous to *tapas*, self-discipline is often at the heart of the virtuosity of musicians, athletes, academics, politicians, and others. Developing exceptional abilities in a whole spectrum of human endeavors is dependent upon people sacrificing time and energy to their chosen activity. Professional musicians and athletes spend innumerable hours in repetitive training, often throughout their entire career or lifetime. Even with an exceptional amount of raw talent—such as a musical "ear" or physical size, speed, and agility—performing at an elite level requires a high degree of training. Though many aspire to the heights of performance, few are ready to make the types of sacrifices called for. It can be inspiring to watch highly trained athletes and musicians perform, and for many people in our contemporary society there is great devotion to spectacles like concerts or athletic events. Often those who have sacrificed the most in their personal lives are the ones who reach the upper echelons or levels of their chosen career or discipline. Yet we would again make a mistake to think that the virtuosity or mastery that these figures exhibit is equivalent to spiritual or moral accomplishment. It may indeed be the case that the two can be found together in some instances. We can all think of athletes or musicians, for example, who clearly demonstrate commitment to transforming their world in positive ways in addition to their talent on the field or stage. However, we can all also think of figures of great virtuosity who exemplify the mastery of a particular art or sport and have fallen from the heights when their questionable moral choices in life come to light and are at odds with the image of perfection projected onto them. The point here is that self-discipline can be a source of accomplishment or perfection that is in service of spiritual development, but that is not always the case.

We might also look at the use of herbs (*auṣadhi*) in a similar light. If we consider how our society uses herbs or drugs for accomplishment or to push the boundaries of embodiment, numerous examples come to mind. One is the use of performance-enhancing substances in athletics, which is a clear attempt to reach or transcend the limits of the human body in order to perform at a superior level. This might be compared with the use of attention-deficit medications among scholars and scientists who utilize such substances to extend their ability to focus on a project for extended periods of time and thereby become more productive. Major medications are available to enhance sexual performance, principally for men. Along with the widespread use of caffeine-containing beverages, all sorts of energy drinks and various herbal supplements promise the ability to control and enhance one's energy levels. Psychogenic substances provide access to experiences of altered perception and a range of states of consciousness that have significant differences from ordinary waking consciousness. Some lead to the experience of ecstasy and result in novel ways of viewing the world. All of these examples demonstrate human-performance augmentation.

It should be noted that the use of herbs as a spiritual practice also differs from the *aṣṭāṅgayoga* system to the degree that taking an herb or other substance does not require physical and psychological preparation. To put it another way, *aṣṭāṅgayoga* is a systematic discipline of yoga in which the practitioner builds up a practice over a period of time, advancing in the practice as the body and mind develop skills and stamina. A potential risk of using herbs or drugs to enhance physical or mental performance is that they can sap the resources of the mind and body, especially if one is not prepared for the energetic level of a particular activity, and lead to physical and psychological trauma. This type of functional imbalance may increase with continued use and make such practices unsustainable, if not outright damaging, over time. Also, to the degree that yogic realization requires clarity of mind, the use of herbs or drugs that obscure the mind or warp perception in some way will be counterproductive in the end.

Lastly, the use of incantation (*mantra*) as a means to accomplishment in the world is evident in the contemporary context in numerous ways. In addition to being an important part of establishing authority in contemporary Hindu traditions, *mantra* can be said to refer to a broader spectrum of human experience. In particular, it is coextensive with larger notions of the mastery of speech, especially the building blocks of language, text, and literature that underpin human communication. This is exemplified, for example, in the highly refined forms of speech found in the world of politics. The emotive and stylistic force, or rhetorical force, exemplified in the power of political speech and language demonstrates words' ability to evoke profound emotion and to act as driving forces in the way that we construct our view of the world and our place in it. Likewise, the language of law undergirds society in a range of ways, and those who master its subtleties wield significant power and influence. As with our previous examples, control over the power of speech is morally and spiritually ambiguous. Powerful speech is not unique to individuals who are morally or spiritually developed. Many of us are skeptical of the intentions of politicians, for example, even if they are able to speak compellingly and articulately. We can also contemplate the moral ambivalence of control over the language of law, which can be wielded in support of a very wide range of interests. Popular musical vocalists might also be considered to have a certain degree of power over their listeners as the result of their performative abilities, regardless of the content of their message. Having power over the capacity of speech may indeed give individuals power in the world, but such power does not equal spiritual or moral accomplishment.

The mastery of *saṃyama*—the obtaining of powers—is a logical extension of the process of mastery that we have seen at all levels of the *aṣṭāṅgayoga*. *Saṃyama* is a discipline of "pattern watching" that yields insight into some aspect of one's embodiment or the world. In the case of *samādhi*, mastering the dynamism of the mind yields perceptual capabilities that can be applied, in principle, to any worldly object. The coherence of the eight limbs is exemplified in the harmonious relationship between them and the movement toward subtle modes of perception and action from less refined ones.

Kaivalya

In the yoga philosophy, the final goal of *aṣṭāṅgayoga* is the attainment of *kaivalya*, or liberation. *Kaivalya* occurs when the *yogin* or *yoginī* is able to meditatively discern that the power of consciousness is distinct from the operations of the mind and body. When the yogic disciplines of the eight limbs are perfected and the modifications of the mind cease, it becomes evident that the mind is not, in fact, the real person and that consciousness is a nonlocalized awareness that is reflected through the mind. This is understood to be a deep and existential realization of the coextensive nature of mind and body, and the distinct reality of consciousness. *Kaivalya* is sometimes equated with *para-vairāgya*, which is the idea of detachment or dispassion, a state of complete equanimity or peace with respect to the turnings of the world. These two aspects are fundamentally intertwined. The principal cause of attachment and misery in the world is said to be none other than a deep-seated conflation of self-identity and ego-identity. In other words, the very motivation for clinging to worldly objects and experiences can be found in the misidentification of one's ultimate self with that of the "I" constituted by the mind and body. If the illusion of ego-identity is dissolved, then afflicted emotions like anger, hatred, jealousy, greed, and so forth do not arise. Throughout the practice of the *aṣṭāṅgayoga* system, one is performing practices that aim at limiting or reducing egocentric agency, thereby bringing the practitioner closer to realizing who he or she really is. One of the subtle but profitable ironies of the yoga philosophy is that the very things that bind us to misery can also become the basis for our liberation.

In some interpretations of the yoga philosophy, *kaivalya* is viewed as a final withdrawal from the world. This places emphasis on the idea of *kaivalya* as "aloneness." However, many interpreters of the yoga philosophy assert that *kaivalya* is only the beginning of the story, rather than the end. The *yogin* or *yoginī* who has reached *kaivalya* is no longer caught up in the false identification of the self with his or her transitory mind or body. However, the same world that binds a person can be an instrument for self-knowledge and thus liberation. Though the world ceases to be what it once was for the liberated *yogin* or *yoginī*, it still exists for others. Therefore, skillful participation in the world for the sake of others remains as a possibility for those who have untangled themselves from it. This can be compared to the notion of Īśvara, who is viewed as a person who is not caught up in the world and chooses to manifest in the world in order to pass the knowledge of yoga on to others. Hindu narrative literature contains themes regarding the yoga adept who is "liberated in life" (*jīvanmukti*), who uses his or her yoga-born powers in a spirit of playful assistance to others—such as through teaching and even through composing poetry. This is quite similar in many respects to Buddhist conceptions of enlightened beings, such as arhats, bodhisattvas, and buddhas, who all are characterized as spiritually awakened beings and spiritual teachers motivated by compassion for the world. Some traditions of yoga see liberation as ultimately merging into a deity or greater being; others emphasize the uniqueness of each liberated being. Nevertheless, all share the understanding that yoga offers a path to transformation that can lead to both spiritual power within the world and liberation from bondage to the world. From the viewpoint of the yoga philosophy, having the first without the second is an inferior path, and one that leads to future misery. The two together, however, are said to offer infinite potential.

6

Integration

YS I.21 *tīvrasaṃvegānām āsannaḥ*

Those of intense zeal are near [to the goal].

As we have discussed in several contexts, one of the underlying themes of yoga is the idea that self-transformation requires consistent effort over time. Though there are moments of insight that may accelerate the process, the foundation of the practice of yoga is a long-term commitment to daily practice. Some yoga teachers will state that the practice of yoga is a process that can extend over many lives, and that, in fact, if a person is practicing yoga now, he or she was likely introduced to it in a former life. One way to view a statement like this is to note how what we have done in the past is reflected in the present and how what we are doing now will reflect into the future. Our actions in the present are seeds of our future life. The decisions we make and actions we take now condition what our future will look like, whether we think of this in terms of one life or many. This is, in principle, what is meant by the term *karma*, which literally means "action."

From the viewpoint of the yoga philosophy, effort is cumulative. The force of an action increases in a manner proportionate to the intensity and frequency of that action. The practice of yoga performed with intensity and frequency becomes fruitful and beneficial quickly. A practice that is not performed with intensity or frequency is like a plant that is not given either appropriate water or appropriate sunlight—it quickly withers away. Developing a yoga practice requires a serious commitment, so that one's practice can grow and thrive. By "serious," we do not mean without humor. In fact, keeping a sense of humor is essential to sustaining a long-term yoga practice and to avoiding dogmatism and burnout. The point is that creating the intention to make yoga a part of everyday life is a gateway to bringing one's practice to a higher level.

One way to explain this depth of commitment in yoga is in terms of developing the yogic principle of faith or confidence (*śraddhā*). For many people, the idea of faith brings to mind a blind adherence to some dogmatic or authoritarian belief that is not grounded in individual experience. What we are referring to here might therefore be better described as confidence, in that it refers to the idea of testing what one learns in the laboratory of one's own experience—and building confidence in what rings true and is transformative. It also means not merely dabbling in something but rather investing the time and energy necessary to evaluate it properly. In one of the contemporary Tibetan traditions of Buddhist meditation, for example, in order to build one's motivation and dedication to meditation, a practitioner is first directed to contemplate its potential benefits, and, in principle, as one begins to experience such benefits, confidence grows and further motivates continued practice, creating a feedback loop.

Building a commitment to practice and the intensity and continuity necessary to grow in one's practice of yoga plays out in two ways. The first way is in terms of formal practice, which includes self-study and the commitment to formal training. Self-study is often the first step in developing a practice of yoga, typically drawing upon books and multimedia sources. This is typically expanded and deepened by a commitment to formal training with a particular teacher or within a particular school or tradition of yoga. Traditional sources often emphasize the idea of committing oneself to a teacher or guru for the sake of obtaining authoritative knowledge from someone who embodies the truth of the tradition through their own experience of applying the teaching. The challenge is to find an authentic and skilled teacher who approaches teaching with integrity and responsibility. As we have discussed, it is not unheard of for individuals to use their impressive degree of mastery of the practice of yoga for the purpose of pursuing power, wealth, sex, and other mundane or worldly goods. Committing to long-term study with any yoga tradition or teacher calls for a diligent effort to educate oneself about the given teacher or tradition. Exploring a number of different schools of yoga and spending time with a number of different teachers before committing oneself to a particular type of practice is an approach that increases the likelihood of meeting with success and avoiding pitfalls. It makes a great deal of sense to find a practice that is in harmony with one's needs and values and to apply oneself in a determined way, rather than accepting teachings that don't fit one's situation or that lack substance. One should keep in mind, though, that moving from teacher to teacher without developing depth in one's practice is unlikely to provide the sort of stable and habit-driven practice that is so essential to success in yoga.

The second way that the commitment to intensity and continuity in yoga practice plays out is in terms of the integration of yoga into everyday life. On one level, a regular yoga practice almost inescapably changes the nature of one's everyday life in the world. The peace and tranquillity, as well as the health benefits, that one draws from practice undoubtedly impact one's everyday experience. Another dimension of this is the way in which we can consciously make our everyday experiences a practice of yoga in and of themselves. As we discussed earlier, one may try to cultivate the limbs of yoga in the midst of one's everyday responsibilities and activities, whether in work, parenting, daily chores, hobbies, or athletic activities, for example. This is to ask the question, how can we draw the eight limbs of yoga into our lives and ultimately transform all that we do, pleasant or painful, into a contemplative exercise? We can also examine the ways in which the lifestyle choices we are making are working either in harmony with or counter to our practice of yoga. We may ask ourselves how we might enhance or expand the activities that strengthen our yoga practice and how we might cut back or eliminate the activities that are at odds with it. Buddhist traditions refer to the concept of "right livelihood," which similarly forwards the idea that how we make our way in the world should be consistent with our moral and spiritual aspirations.

It makes sense to scale back the intensity of one's practice at certain times, such as following an injury, during illness, or when one has become exhausted. Learning to modulate and adjust one's efforts to fit the present conditions of one's life is an extremely important part of the practice of yoga. However, a baseline of commitment, enthusiasm, and discipline is at the heart of a successful yoga practice, even in times of adversity.

The eight limbs of yoga provide tools and inspiration for establishing and cultivating a fruitful and rewarding practice of yoga. They are simple and yet profound, offering a formulation of yoga that is eminently useful in daily yoga practice and in everyday life.

> May we all find success in our efforts to transform ourselves and bring more peace and compassion to the world through the practice of yoga.

Suggested Reading

TRANSLATIONS OF THE *YOGASŪTRA*

Āraṇya, Hariharānanda. *Yoga Philosophy of Patañjali: Containing His Yoga Aphorisms with Vyāsa's Commentary in Sanskrit and a Translation with Annotations Including Many Suggestions for the Practice of Yoga.* Translated by P. N. Mukerji. Albany: State University of New York Press, 1983.

Arya, Pandit Usharbudh. *Yoga-Sūtras of Patañjali with the Exposition of Vyāsa: A Translation and Commentary.* Vol. 1, *Samādhipāda.* Honesdale, Penn.: Himalayan Institute Press, 1986.

Bryant, Edwin F. *The Yoga Sūtras of Patañjali: A New Edition, Translation, and Commentary; With Insights from the Traditional Commentators.* New York: North Point Press, 2009.

Chapple, Christopher Key. *Yoga and the Luminous: Patañjali's Spiritual Path to Freedom.* Albany: State University of New York Press, 2008.

Feuerstein, Georg. *The Yoga-Sūtra of Patañjali: A New Translation and Commentary.* Rochester, Vt.: Inner Traditions International, 1989.

Rukmani, T. S. *Yogavārttika of Vijñānabhikṣu.* New Delhi: Munshiram Manoharlal Publishers, 1998–2007.

Stoler Miller, Barbara, trans. *Yoga: Discipline of Freedom; The Yoga Sutra Attributed to Patanjali.* Berkeley: University of California Press, 1996.

Veda Bharati, Swami. *Yoga Sūtras of Patañjali with the Exposition of Vyāsa: A Translation and Commentary.* Vol. 2, *Sadhānapāda.* Delhi: Motilal Banarsidass Publishers, 2004.

TRANSLATIONS OF HAṬHAYOGA TEXTS

Aiyangar, M. Srinivasa. *The Haṭhayogapradīpikā of Svātmārāma: With the Commentary Jyotsnā of Brahmānanda and English Translation.* Madras: Adyar Library and Research Centre, 1972.

Akers, Brian Dana. *The Hatha Yoga Pradipika.* Woodstock, N.Y.: YogaVidya, 2002.

Bhatt, G. P., ed. *The Forceful Yoga: Being the Translation of Haṭhayoga-Pradīpikā, Gheraṇḍa-Saṃhitā and Śiva-Saṃhitā.* Translated by Pancham Sinh and Srisa Chandra Vasu. Delhi: Motilal Banarsidass Publishers, 2009.

Mallinson, James. *The Gheranda Samhita: The Original Sanskrit.* Woodstock, N.Y.: YogaVidya, 2004.

HISTORICAL AND PHILOSOPHICAL STUDY OF YOGA AND TANTRIC TRADITIONS

Bühnemann, Gudrun. *Eighty-four Asanas in Yoga: A Survey of Traditions, with Illustrations.* New Delhi: D.K. Printworld, 2007.

Burley, Mikel. *Haṭha-Yoga: Its Context, Theory, and Practice.* Delhi: Motilal Banarsidass Publishers, 2000.

Connolly, Peter. *A Student's Guide to the History and Philosophy of Yoga.* London: Equinox, 2007.

De Michelis, Elizabeth. *A History of Modern Yoga: Patañjali and Western Esotericism.* London: Continuum, 2005.

Eliade, Mircea. *Yoga: Immortality and Freedom.* Princeton: Princeton University Press, 2009.

Feuerstein, Georg. *The Philosophy of Classical Yoga.* Rochester, Vt.: Inner Traditions, 1996.

———. *Tantra: Path of Ecstasy.* Boston: Shambhala, 1998.

———. *Yoga: The Technology of Ecstasy.* Los Angeles: JP Tarcher, 1989.

———. *The Yoga Tradition: Its History, Literature, Philosophy, and Practice.* Prescott, Ariz.: Hohm Press, 1998.

Gunaratana, Henepola. *The Path of Serenity and Insight: An Explanation of the Buddhist Jhānas.* Delhi: Motilal Banarsidass Publishers, 1985.

Jacobsen, Knut A. *Theory and Practice of Yoga: Essays in Honour of Gerald James Larson.* Leiden: Brill, 2011.

———. *Yoga Powers: Extraordinary Capacities Attained Through Meditation and Concentration.* Vol. 37. Leiden: Brill, 2011.

Larson, Gerald James, and Ram Shankar Bhattacharya. *Encyclopedia of Indian Philosophies.* Vol. 12, *Yoga: India's Philosophy of Meditation.* Delhi: Motilal Banarsidass Publishers, 2008.

Love, Robert. *The Great Oom: The Improbable Birth of Yoga in America*. New York: Viking, 2010.

Phillips, Stephen H. *Yoga, Karma, and Rebirth: A Brief History and Philosophy*. New York: Columbia University Press, 2009.

Ray, Reginald A. *Secret of the Vajra World: The Tantric Buddhism of Tibet*. Boston: Shambhala, 2001.

Samuel, Geoffrey. *The Origins of Yoga and Tantra: Indic Religions to the Thirteenth Century*. New York: Cambridge University Press, 2008.

Sarbacker, Stuart Ray. *Samādhi: The Numinous and Cessative in Indo-Tibetan Yoga*. Albany: State University of New York Press, 2005.

Shaw, Sarah. *Buddhist Meditation: An Anthology of Texts from the Pali Canon*. London: Routledge, 2006.

Singleton, Mark. *Yoga Body: The Origins of Modern Posture Practice*. Oxford: Oxford University Press, 2010.

Singleton, Mark, and Jean Byrne. *Yoga in the Modern World: Contemporary Perspectives*. London: Routledge, 2008.

Singleton, Mark, and Ellen Goldberg. *Gurus of Modern Yoga*. Oxford: Oxford University Press, 2013.

Syman, Stefanie. *The Subtle Body: The Story of Yoga in America*. New York: Farrar, Straus and Giroux, 2010.

Whicher, Ian. *The Integrity of the Yoga Darsana: A Reconsideration of Classical Yoga*. Albany: State University of New York Press, 1998.

White, David Gordon. *Sinister Yogis*. Chicago: University of Chicago Press, 2009.

———. *Tantra in Practice*. Princeton: Princeton University Press, 2000.

———. *Yoga in Practice*. Princeton: Princeton University Press, 2012.

MODERN YOGA PHILOSOPHY AND PRACTICE

Desikachar, T.K.V. *The Heart of Yoga: Developing a Personal Practice*. Rochester, Vt.: Inner Traditions, 1999.

Freeman, Richard. *The Mirror of Yoga: Awakening the Intelligence of Body and Mind*. Boston: Shambhala, 2010.

Iyengar, B.K.S. *Core of the Yoga Sutras: The Definitive Guide to the Philosophy of Yoga*. London: HarperThorsons, 2012.

———. *Light on Prānāyāma: The Yogic Art of Breathing*. New York: Crossroad, 1981.

———. *Light on Yoga: Yoga Dīpikā*. New York: Schocken Books, 1979.

Jois, Sri. K. Pattabhi. *Yoga Mala: The Original Teachings of Ashtanga Yoga Master Sri. K. Pattabhi Jois*. New York: North Point Press, 2002.

Ramaswami, Srivatsa. *Yoga for the Three Stages of Life: Developing Your Practice as an Art Form, a Physical Therapy, and a Guiding Philosophy*. Rochester, Vt.: Inner Traditions, 2000.

Rosen, Richard. *Original Yoga: Rediscovering Traditional Practices of Hatha Yoga*. Boston: Shambhala, 2012.

Stone, Michael. *Awake in the World: Teachings from Yoga & Buddhism for Living an Engaged Life*. Boston: Shambhala, 2011.

———. *Freeing the Body, Freeing the Mind: Writings on the Connections Between Yoga and Buddhism*. Boston: Shambhala, 2010.

———. *The Inner Tradition of Yoga: A Guide to Yoga Philosophy for the Contemporary Practitioner*. Boston: Shambhala, 2008.

———. *Yoga for a World Out of Balance: Teachings on Ethics and Social Action*. Boston: Shambhala, 2009.

BUDDHIST MEDITATION AND MINDFULNESS PRACTICES

Bhikkhu, Buddhadasa. *Mindfulness of Breathing: A Manual for Serious Beginners*. Boston: Wisdom, 2007.

Brahm, Ajahn. *Mindfulness, Bliss, and Beyond: A Meditator's Handbook*. Boston: Wisdom, 2006.

Catherine, Shaila. *Focused and Fearless: A Meditator's Guide to States of Deep Joy, Calm, and Clarity*. Boston: Wisdom, 2008.

———. *Wisdom Wide and Deep: A Practical Handbook for Mastering Jhana and Vipassana*. Boston: Wisdom, 2011.

Gunaratana, Henepola. *Mindfulness in Plain English*. Boston: Wisdom, 2002.

Gyatso, Tenzin (XIV Dalai Lama). *How to Expand Love: Widening the Circle of Loving Relationships*. New York: Atria, 2005.

———. *Opening the Eye of New Awareness*. Boston: Wisdom, 2009.

Kabat-Zinn, Jon. *Coming to Our Senses: Healing Ourselves and the World Through Mindfulness*. New York: Hyperion, 2005.

Kabat-Zinn, Jon, and University of Massachusetts Medical Center/Worcester Stress Reduction Clinic. *Full Catastrophe Living: Using the Wisdom of Your Body and Mind to Face Stress, Pain, and Illness*. New York: Delacorte Press, 1990.

Nhat Hanh, Thich. *The Miracle of Mindfulness: An Introduction to the Practice of Meditation*. Boston: Beacon, 1999.

———. *Teachings on Love*. Berkeley: Parallax Press, 2007.

———. *True Love: A Practice for Awakening the Heart*. Boston: Shambhala, 2011.

Snyder, Stephen, and Tina Rasmussen. *Practicing the Jhānas: Traditional Concen-*

tration Meditation as Presented by the Venerable Pa Auk Sayadaw. Boston: Shambhala, 2009.

Wangyal, Tenzin. *Awakening the Luminous Mind: Tibetan Meditation for Peace and Joy*. New York: Hay House, 2012.

———. *Awakening the Sacred Body: Tibetan Yogas of Breath and Movement*. New York: Hay House, 2011.

———. *Tibetan Sound Healing: Seven Guided Practices to Clear Obstacles, Cultivate Positive Qualities, and Uncover Your Inherent Wisdom*. Boulder, Colo.: Sounds True, 2011.

Zahler, Leah. *Meditative States in Tibetan Buddhism*. Boston: Wisdom, 1997.

Acknowledgments

This book is the product of a spirit of engagement with life and an active examination of the relationship that is shared between the authors and our families, friends, colleagues, and teachers. We could not have written this without the support of a network of people around us who, on various levels, sympathize with our experiments in yoga. Our families have provided an ongoing source of support and inspiration throughout this process, reminding us of the need to ground our ideas in the "real world" experience of daily life. Our friends have also played important roles in helping us develop our ideas, often through late-night conversations and jam sessions. Our academic colleagues and fellow yoga practitioners have helped create a supportive laboratory context in which we have striven to develop our ideas and our practices. Lastly, we wish to acknowledge the collective efforts of our many teachers, whose instruction continues to help us grow into more kind, compassionate, and peaceful human beings. We hope that any fraction of their inspiration and light shines through in this work.

Stuart would especially like to thank his loving and

fierce partner, Sara Zeman, and his daughters, Tara and Stella Sarbacker; his parents, John and Margaret Sarbacker; his friends and compatriots Richard Miller and Michael Baker; his friends and colleagues in the School of History, Philosophy, and Religion at Oregon State University; his friends, faculty, and students from the Eugene School of Yoga, especially Kevin Kimple and Dan Cox; and his many mentors and teachers, including Chris Chapple, Ian Whicher, Gerald Larson, Indira Junghare, T. S. Rukmani, David Knipe, John Dunne, Sriram Agashe, and Manju Jois, among many others.

Kevin would like to thank Richard Freeman, to whom he is forever grateful for tolerating his incessant shout-outs and interruptions, for splitting his head wide open and demonstrating how deep the exploration of yoga and relationship can really go, and for leading his way to his studies with Sri K. Pattabhi Jois, who insisted that he always practice through his fears and many "bad thoughts." To Guruji, his deepest thanks for instilling in him the faith that he simply needed to keep practicing and everything else would fall into place. Thanks also to Raymond Hill, his high school principal, who devoted his life to his students and created the context for so many to flourish, and David Wood, who saved him from imminent self-destruction and taught him to dance through life. Kevin sends all his love to his son, Kirpal, whose very presence reminds him daily of what is truly important. Lastly, he thanks all in the great lineage of teachers.

We both would like to thank the eminent yoga author Stefanie Syman for encouraging us to bring the project to FSG; Katie Van Heest at Tweed Editing, who helped bring a shine to the book in the final stages of writing and editing; and Jeff Seroy at FSG, whose adventurous spirit has played a key role in bringing the project to fruitful completion.